100 Questions & Answers About Your Child's OCD

Josiane Cobert, MD

Child and Adolescent Psychiatrist
Hospital-Based Practice
Elizabeth, NJ

JONES AND BARTLETT PUBLISHERS

Sudbury, Massachusetts

BOSTON   TORONTO   LONDON   SINGAPORE

World Headquarters

Jones and Bartlett Publishers	Jones and Bartlett Publishers	Jones and Bartlett Publishers
40 Tall Pine Drive	Canada	International
Sudbury, MA 01776	6339 Ormindale Way	Barb House, Barb Mews
978-443-5000	Mississauga, Ontario L5V 1J2	London W6 7PA
info@jbpub.com	Canada	United Kingdom
www.jbpub.com		

Jones and Bartlett's books and products are available through most bookstores and online booksellers. To contact Jones and Bartlett Publishers directly, call 800-832-0034, fax 978-443-8000, or visit our website, www.jbpub.com.

Substantial discounts on bulk quantities of Jones and Bartlett's publications are available to corporations, professional associations, and other qualified organizations. For details and specific discount information, contact the special sales department at Jones and Bartlett via the above contact information or send an email to specialsales@jbpub.com.

The authors, editor, and publisher have made every effort to provide accurate information. However, they are not responsible for errors, omissions, or for any outcomes related to the use of the contents of this book and take no responsibility for the use of the products and procedures described. Treatments and side effects described in this book may not be applicable to all people; likewise, some people may require a dose or experience a side effect that is not described herein. Drugs and medical devices are discussed that may have limited availability controlled by the Food and Drug Administration (FDA) for use only in a research study or clinical trial. Research, clinical practice, and government regulations often change the accepted standard in this field. When consideration is being given to use of any drug in the clinical setting, the healthcare provider or reader is responsible for determining FDA status of the drug, reading the package insert, and reviewing prescribing information for the most up-to-date recommendations on dose, precautions, and contraindications, and determining the appropriate usage for the product. This is especially important in the case of drugs that are new or seldom used.

Production Credits

Executive Publisher: Christopher Davis
Senior Acquisitions Editor: Alison Hankey
Production Editor: Rachel Rossi
Senior Editorial Assistant: Jessica Acox
Marketing Manager: Ilana Goddess

VP, Manufacturing and Inventory Control:
  Therese Connell
Composition: Appingo Publishing Services
Printing and Binding: Malloy, Inc.
Cover Printing: Malloy, Inc.

Cover Credits

Cover Design: Carolyn Downer
Cover Images: Smiling sisters, © Yuri Arcurs/ShutterStock, Inc.; Family portrait, © Dmitriy Shironosov/Dreamstime.com; Smiling toddler, © Shupian/Dreamstime.com

Library of Congress Cataloging-in-Publication Data
Cobert, Josiane.
  100 questions and answers about your child's obsessive compulsive disorder / Josiane Cobert and Barton Cobert.
    p. cm.
  ISBN-13: 978-0-7637-7154-6 (alk. paper)
  ISBN-10: 0-7637-7154-6 (alk. paper)
  1. Obsessive-compulsive disorder in children—Popular works. I. Cobert, Barton L. II. Title. III. Title: One hundred questions and answers about your child's obsessive compulsive disorder.
  RJ506.O25C65 2010
  618.92'85227--dc22
                              2009001084
6048

Printed in the United States of America
13 12 11 10 09   10 9 8 7 6 5 4 3 2 1

To my children: Emilie and Julien

CONTENTS

Since you are reading this book you are well aware that OCD can be a devastating problem not just for your child but for you and the rest of your family as well as friends, associates, schoolmates and even your employer if caring for your child interferes with work.

You also are likely to have a fairly good understanding of OCD and the issues and treatments associated with it, afterall this is something you live with on a 24/7 basis.

The aim of this little book is to fill in some of the gaps in your knowledge of the disease using a user-friendly format: namely a question and answer session between you and your child's doctor, counselor, health care provider and others involved in his or her care. This is not a textbook but rather a summary of what is known about diagnosis, causes (briefly), treatment, prognosis, and ongoing experimental work. It is purposely kept simple, straightforward and non-technical. If you want further, more detailed information the literary and online references offered in the appendix will be useful.

OCD can cover a broad spectrum ranging from mild to severe, isolated or accompanying other psychiatric diseases in a child. There are no hard-and-fast rules, and predictions are sometimes hard to make about the course of the disease. Nonetheless, over the last 20 years, the understanding of OCD (and of psychiatric diseases in general) has advanced. New treatments (involving both medications and behavioral therapy) have evolved and become available. There is more understanding (and hopefully tolerance) in the community and in the schools for children with OCD. The picture then is guardedly optimistic. The child with OCD can be helped and can live a successful and happy life (as can the family!).

I hope this book will be a small piece of the evolution in the successful treatment of your child with OCD.

PART ONE

The Basics of OCD

What is obsessive-compulsive disorder?

Are OCD symptoms always the same in an individual patient, or do they change over time?

What is the cause of OCD?

More . . .

1. What is obsessive-compulsive disorder?

Obsessions

Recurrent and persistent thoughts, impulses, or images that are experienced as intrusive and inappropriate and that cause marked anxiety or distress.

Compulsions

Repetitive behaviors or mental acts that a person feels driven to perform in response to an obsession, or according to internal rules that must be applied rigidly.

The children may be aware that what they are doing does not make sense, but, nonetheless, they feel very distressed if they do not carry out the compulsions.

There is strong evidence that obsessive-compulsive disorder (OCD) is an illness with a large biological component. OCD is partly due to medical issues (i.e., biological or genetic) and is not just a "mental problem." It is a chronic illness with waxing and waning symptoms.

OCD is a type of anxiety disorder characterized by recurrent **obsessions**, recurrent **compulsions**, or both. Compulsions are also called **rituals** (but not in the religious sense of the word).

Of course, all children have occasional worries and doubts. But when they cannot stop thinking about these concerns, and when these issues start affecting their daily functioning and interfering with others in the family, then this becomes a problem that needs to be addressed.

The children (depending on their age and degree of understanding) may be aware that what they are doing does not make sense, but, nonetheless, they feel very distressed if they do not carry out the compulsions. They want to get rid of the corresponding obsessions. Sometimes these rituals are done to prevent a terrible imagined event from actually happening, and the children feel personally responsible for performing these actions so that nothing bad happens.

The compulsive act is an attempt to decrease the anxiety brought by the obsessive thought. However, it is not always successful, and the anxiety might even increase.

Obsession → Anxiety → Compulsion → Anxiety relief (transient)

2. Is OCD common, or are we just unlucky?

OCD is quite common. It afflicts about 1 million children in the United States. It is the fourth most frequent psychiatric disorder after **phobias**, substance abuse, and major depressive disorders.

There is no clear agreement over the actual number of people with OCD. This lack of agreement is due to the variations in how the studies were conducted and in how the researchers made the diagnosis of OCD. In any case, roughly 1% of people in the U.S. population have OCD. Many researchers feel the correct value may be 2 or 3 times higher. Overall, it appears that OCD is more prevalent now than it was in the 1950s.

OCD tends to be underdiagnosed and undertreated for many reasons. Some people may not have access to treatment resources. Others are ashamed of their symptoms and are very secretive about them. Some people do not understand that it is an illness that can be treated, and they do not seek treatment. Many health providers are not familiar with the symptoms and have not been trained to provide the appropriate treatment. There is also a large proportion of people who have mild (sub-threshold) symptoms that are, nevertheless, noticeable.

OCD in children is usually diagnosed between 7 and 12 years of age. During this period, children are becoming more involved with their peers, and they can notice that they behave differently and feel more distressed.

Many children younger than 6 years old have frequent urges to make things "just right" and have preoccupations with symmetry and rules. These concerns usually decrease with age and do not become OCD. For example, one study showed that nearly two-thirds of fourth graders reported preoccupations with guilt about lying and were engaging in checking behaviors (e.g., looking multiple times to see if the door really is closed or if the object they just put in a particular place is really in the right place). In the same study, half of the

Ritual

A repetitive, systematic behavioral process enacted to neutralize or prevent anxiety; a symptom of obsessive-compulsive disorder (OCD).

Phobia

An objectively unfounded, morbid dread or fear that arouses a state of panic.

The Basics of OCD

same age group also reported fears about contamination and germs. By eighth grade, rates for these concerns decreased to 40%. However, 60% of eighth graders reported worries about cleanliness, and 50% had intrusive unpleasant or even nasty thoughts. So, while having such thoughts and ideas does not necessarily mean OCD will develop, children with more symptoms and high anxiety might represent a group at risk to develop OCD.

3. OCD started in my son at 5 years of age. Is this unusual? What age does it usually start at? Is it only a childhood disease? Is it different in boys than in girls?

One-third to one-half of adults with OCD say their symptoms started before they were 15 years old. Most males report an onset between 6 and 15 years of age. Women, however, may have a later onset of symptoms, typically between 20 and 30 years of age. One report has indicated that the average age when a patient seeks medical help is about 27 years old.

These figures indicate that OCD is by no means limited to children and that adults suffer from this problem too. It is unfortunate that many people wait until they are adults before seeking treatment even though the problems started in their childhood. The average time between the onset of symptoms and appropriate treatment is about 17 years in adults.

The symptoms of OCD often appear insidiously in children and can be mistaken for behavioral difficulties; for instance, a child may be called disobedient for refusing to do a chore when in fact the child has fears of contamination. Diagnosis can be very tricky, particularly if there are other medical or psychiatric comorbid conditions. In other children, OCD symptoms may suddenly appear "overnight."

Males and females are equally affected (i.e., there is an equal **prevalence** between males and females). However, boys often

Prevalence

The total number of cases of a disease in a population at a particular point in time. This number includes new and old cases.

have an earlier onset of the disease. Symptoms are present an average of 5 to 8 years before patients reach medical attention, and male patients tend to have a longer duration of the illness before they seek treatment.

In general, the disease is the same in males and females. However, premenstrual worsening of OCD symptoms occurs in 20% to 40% of women with OCD. Many women identify the onset of their disease as having occurred when they became pregnant.

4. Are there differences between OCD that starts in childhood and OCD that starts in adulthood and do they both ever go away?

Yes, there are important clinical differences between OCD that starts in childhood and OCD that starts in adulthood. Childhood OCD has been associated with more severe symptoms and more compulsions, and it is frequently associated with other psychiatric disorders such as ADHD, **tic** disorders, and multiple anxiety disorders.

If the early onset cases are first treated during adulthood, there is frequently a poor response to the medications.

OCD may not go away on its own. If not treated, OCD can become a long-term disorder. Some older studies, done before effective medicines were available, showed that about three-fourths of adult patients had a chronic and continuous course with waxing and waning symptoms. Of those patients, two-thirds improved within a decade after the OCD symptoms started, but about 10% had a deteriorating course, and some (up to 25%) had an episodic course with full **remissions** lasting up to 6 months. Sometimes, patients experience only partial remissions. In one study, 17% of subjects had relapses after 20 years of remission. In other words, all patterns are possible, and it cannot be predicted up front which course a particular patient will take.

Remission

When symptoms are reduced to a minimal level, with a Y-BOCS of <16. Recovery and remission are considered high levels of response. See page 47 on Y-BOCS.

The Basics of OCD

5. Are OCD symptoms always the same in an individual patient, or do they change over time?

Your child may have particular obsessions and compulsions now and completely different symptoms during a recurrence. The symptoms frequently change as the child gets older.

They may change. Your child may have particular obsessions and compulsions now and completely different symptoms during a recurrence. The symptoms frequently change as the child gets older. No one is sure why. For example, a young child may worry about developing a serious illness or about intruders entering the house or about a parent dying. A 6- or 7-year-old child may worry about germs. A 17-year-old adolescent may worry about fires or getting "crazy." A child may move from one set of worries to another over time. These symptoms may completely disappear with treatment. But, later on, even as an adult, if the OCD reappears, it might be with completely different obsessions, such as doubting what he or she has just done and reorganizing a task that was just done multiple times.

6. What are the costs of OCD?

There are significant costs both to the individual patient and family, and to society at large. OCD impairs the patient's quality of life. Children with moderate to severe OCD who are not being treated with medication have worse social functioning and performance. The more severe the symptoms, the more impaired the social functioning is. Children may have fewer friends and may not be able to perform appropriately in school and in extra-curricular activities. They may suffer from low self-esteem. There is also a lower likelihood of adult OCD patients getting married.

Family members suffer as well. OCD patients may create disharmony by being excessively dependent on family members or by taking up space in the home if they are hoarders and accumulate unnecessary objects. Parents may have difficulty taking holidays with their OCD children; they may be concerned about how people outside of the close family will judge or tolerate them, or they may be too preoccupied with their children to enjoy leisure activities. All of this produces significant stress on the family.

There are high social costs, as OCD in adulthood may interfere with patients' work. In 1990, the estimated direct costs of OCD to the U.S. economy were $2.1 billion, and the indirect costs (lost productivity) were about $6.2 billion. High social costs are reflected by high rates of unemployment, disability, and welfare payments.

7. Is OCD hereditary? What are the chances that my child will inherit OCD if someone in the family has it already? Is it contagious? Is it more common in some groups of people than in others?

There is strong evidence that genetic transmission of OCD exists in some people.

Some forms of OCD may be hereditary. In identical twins (same egg), there is a higher rate of OCD in both siblings than in non-identical twins (different eggs). Higher rates of OCD are seen among first-degree relatives of patients who have OCD. One study found that in the parents of children with OCD, 10% had OCD themselves, and another 25% had milder symptoms of obsessions and compulsions. Another study found that if OCD begins at an earlier age, there is a greater likelihood of OCD among relatives. It is believed that the tendency toward anxiety might also be hereditary.

In patients who have **Tourette syndrome** with or without OCD, there is an increased rate of OCD in family members. Tourette syndrome is a disease characterized by **motor tics** (i.e., abnormal repetitive muscle movements such as winking) and **vocal tics** such as grunts or explosive sounds. The prevalence of these two disorders within families suggests that some cases of OCD may be tied genetically to Tourette syndrome. There are, however, many cases of OCD where there are no other family members with OCD or any other psychiatric disease.

OCD frequently runs in families. However, it appears that genes are only partially responsible for causing OCD. If OCD

Tourette syndrome

A disorder characterized by numerous motor and vocal tics. To be diagnosed with Tourette syndrome, tics must be present for at least 1 year.

Vocal tics:

Involuntary sounds such as throat clearing, sniffing, or words.

Autosomal dominant transmission

In genetics and heredity, a trait that needs to be in only one parent to be transmitted to the offspring.

Serotonin

A neurotransmitter that may be decreased in depression and panic attacks.

Dopamine

A hormone and neurotransmitter. Dopamine cannot cross the blood–brain barrier; thus, when given as a drug, it does not directly affect the central nervous system.

Glutamate

Glutamate is the most abundant excitatory neurotransmitter in the mammalian nervous system. Because of its role in synaptic plasticity, it is believed that glutamic acid is involved in cognitive functions like learning and memory in the brain.

were only due to the genes, in pairs of identical twins, both siblings would have it. But this is not always the case. Other factors are involved. Some researchers believe that a viral infection or exposure to an environmental toxin may be the cause or the trigger for OCD, separate from genetics and family history. It has also been noted that children who develop OCD are more likely to have blood relatives with OCD than those who develop OCD as adults. As we have seen, there may be different types of OCD, some inherited and some not.

Here is what we know about the likelihood of genetic transmission:

- If a parent has OCD, the likelihood that the child will be affected is about 2% to 8%. The chances will increase if the parents themselves also have a family history of OCD.
- If the parent has OCD that began in childhood (early onset OCD), the chances of passing on the disorder are increased.
- If there are blood relatives or a family history of tic disorders (such as Tourette syndrome) or anxiety disorders, then the child is probably at greater risk for OCD (and tics or anxiety disorders) than someone without this history.

Evidence exists that OCD can be transmitted in an **autosomal dominant** fashion. The genes involved are related to the **serotonin**, **dopamine**, and **glutamate** neurotransmitter systems.

Although OCD is not contagious, there is some thought that one of the causes of OCD in some children could be streptococcal ("strep") infection—which may produce many diseases, such as sore throat, kidney disease, or heart murmurs. Although such an infection can be spread, the OCD itself cannot be transmitted from one individual to another.

OCD exists in all ethnic groups. Various studies in ethnic groups have not shown any difference in occurrence rates. There are noted differences among ethnic groups, however, in regard to access to health care (particularly mental health care), which may affect diagnosis and treatment of OCD. In addition, there are differences in the way various groups respond to medications. These differences pertain not just to psychiatric medications but to various other drugs, such as those used in treating high blood pressure.

There are some suggestions that religion might play a role in the development of OCD. For some, religious practices may become compulsive, joyless behaviors, and specific obsessions and compulsions may vary according to the individual's religion. Religious faith and religious education are not generally the causes of scrupulosity, which is defined as the excessive concern over one's personal sins and preoccupation with a trivial part of the religious ritual instead of the whole picture.

8. What is the cause of OCD?

There are probably multiple causes of OCD. No specific causes have yet been identified, and OCD may actually be the single way the brain responds to multiple problems. This response is similar to the limited way the intestines may produce diarrhea as a reaction to a variety of problems such as bacterial infections, viruses, parasites, food poisoning, anxiety, and malabsorption.

One thing is clear however: OCD is a biological disease of the brain. Adding to this biological element are various environmental factors that also play a role. So although the exact causes of OCD are not fully understood, a combination of biological and environment factors seem to produce it.

Some of the known causes are listed here. The cause that seems to be best understood relates to biochemical factors.

The Basics of OCD

Anatomic Factors

Injuries to certain regions of the brain can produce OCD symptoms. Conversely, in severe OCD that is unresponsive to regular drugs or other treatments, surgery on a particular part of the brain has produced symptomatic improvement in some of these previously non-responsive patients. There are many clues seen in studies using **computed tomography (CT) scans**, **positron emission tomography (PET) scans**, and **magnetic resonance imaging (MRI)** showing various abnormalities in the **frontal cortex** and other areas in the brain. Some studies have shown increased or decreased metabolic activity in various parts of the brain. Other studies have shown defects in one of the "electrical" circuits that transmits nerve impulses to various other parts of the brain, in particular the cortico-striato-thalamo-cortical circuit. Abnormalities have been found in the prefrontal cortex, which is the decision-making portion of the brain, and in parts of the motor and sensory relay stations in the **thalamus**. (See Figures 1 through 3.)

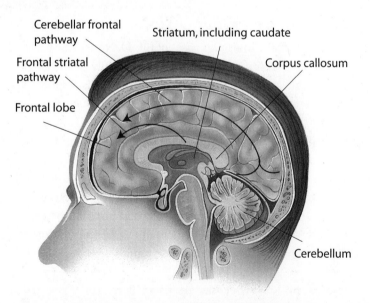

Figure 1   The frontal lobes, the striatum, the cerebellum, and the connections between them are the areas of the brain that are crucial for attention.
SOURCE: Nass, *100 Questions and Answers About Your Child's ADHD*, Jones & Bartlett Publishers, LLC © 2007.

Computed tomography (CT) scan

A form of x-ray that is able to view the brain in more detail than a standard skull x-ray. However, it has been largely replaced by MRI as a diagnostic technique to examine details of the brain. The advantage CT has over MRI is that it detects bone change, whereas MRI views the brain tissue, and is not sensitive to bone.

Positron emission tomography (PET) scan

A test in which a small amount of radioactive glucose (sugar) is injected into a vein, and a scanner is used to make detailed, computerized pictures of areas inside the body (e.g., the brain) where the glucose is used.

Magnetic resonance imaging (MRI)

A technique that creates 3-dimensional images of brain structures using strong magnetic fields. It does not involve x-rays.

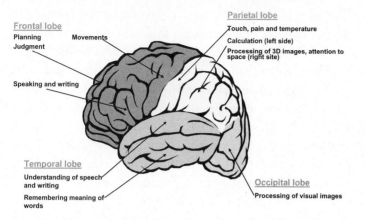

LOCALIZATION OF VARIOUS FUNCTIONS IN HUMAN BRAIN

Figure 2   Localization of Various Functions in the Human Brain
SOURCE: Nass, *100 Questions and Answers About Your Child's ADHD*, Jones & Bartlett Publishers, LLC © 2007.

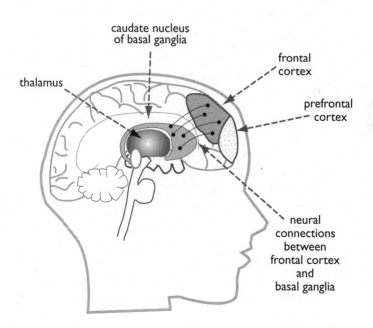

Figure 3   The Brain

Biochemical Factors

The brain is obviously a very complex structure. It contains billions of nerve cells (**neurons**) that must communicate and function well together (Figure 4). They communicate through electrical signals from one nerve cell to the next. Some brain chemicals, called **neurotransmitters**, move the electrical messages from one neuron to another. Neurotransmitters travel from the "end" of one nerve cell (the sending or transmitting cell) to the "beginning" of another cell (the receiving cell) across fluid-filled microscopic spaces between the cells known as **synapses** (Figure 5). To send messages between the cells, neurotransmitters must leave the sending cell, cross the synapse, and bind or attach to a **receptor site** located on the receiving nerve cell. There are many chemicals in the brain that serve this function in the various parts of the brain. In OCD, there are many neurotransmitters that seem to play a role: serotonin, dopamine, glutamate, and possibly others.

Serotonin (also called 5-hydroxytryptamine or 5-HT): Evidence suggests that serotonin is a key element in OCD. Drugs

Neuron

A nerve cell, which is the basic cell unit of the brain and spinal cord. It can send and receive information from other brain cells.

Neurotransmitter

Upon stimulus, a chemical agent that is released by a nerve cell (the presynaptic nerve cell) and travels through the space between that cell and the next nerve cell (synapse) to the postsynaptic cell, where it either stimulates or suppresses that cell. Dopamine, serotonin, and norepinephrine are neurotransmitters.

Synapse

The fluid-filled space between two neurons (brain cells) where neurotransmitters can pass from one cell to the next.

Receptor sites

Places on neurons that bind neurotransmitters or where the medications act. Some medications can increase or decrease the number or sensitivity of receptors.

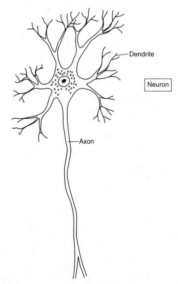

Figure 4   A Neuron

SOURCE: Albrecht, *100 Questions and Answers About Bipolar (Manic Depressive) Disorder*, Jones & Bartlett Publishers, LLC © 2005.

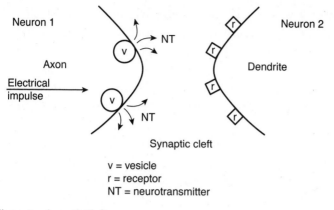

v = vesicle
r = receptor
NT = neurotransmitter

Figure 5   Synaptic Cleft
SOURCE: Albrecht, *100 Questions and Answers About Bipolar (Manic Depressive) Disorder*, Jones & Bartlett Publishers, LLC © 2005.

that affect the serotonin system produce improvements in OCD symptoms. In children receiving drugs that increased the serotonin levels in the brain, certain parts of the brain (e.g., the **caudate** nucleus) that were abnormally large prior to treatment decreased in size, and the OCD symptoms improved.

In OCD, there seems to be a problem either with serotonin levels or with damage at the receptor site in the receiving cells blocking or preventing the serotonin from transmitting the electrical messages. Supporting this idea is the discovery that many OCD patients benefit from the use of a class of medications known to allow more serotonin to reach the receiving nerve cells. These drugs are called **selective serotonin reuptake inhibitors (SSRIs)** and are also effective for the treatment of depression.

Dopamine: Similarly, evidence suggests that dopamine, another neurotransmitter, plays a role in OCD. On brain scans of patients with OCD, there is increased activity in one of the dopamine areas of the brain called the basal ganglia. In patients with known diseases of the basal ganglia, OCD symptoms are frequently present. For example, in patients with Sydenham chorea, brain imaging and spinal fluid studies have shown differences in the neurotransmitter systems between

The Basics of OCD

Caudate

Nucleus within the basal ganglia that is rich in dopamine. It appears to be involved in ADHD, and it is smaller in children with ADHD.

Selective serotonin reuptake inhibitor (SSRI)

A type of antidepressant that does not allow serotonin to be taken up again by neuroreceptors, thereby causing more serotonin to be presented to the neurons, which decreases panic attacks.

patients with OCD and patients with no OCD. Medicines that block dopamine have been used with some success to augment treatment in patients who do not respond well to serotonin drugs only. Thus dopamine too seems to play a role in OCD, and this has led to the use of drugs that work on both the dopamine and serotonin neurotransmitters.

Glutamate: Brain imaging and spinal fluid studies have shown differences in the glutamate system between OCD patients and healthy volunteers. Dysfunction of glutamate neurotransmission has been implicated in the causes of OCD, and recent clinical reports suggest that some drugs that work on glutamate are efficacious in the treatment of this disorder.

Oxytocin: Oxytocin is a hormone that aids in childbirth by increasing during labor and in subsequent breast-feeding. Somewhat surprisingly, it also functions in the brain as a neurotransmitter, having nothing to do there with female reproduction. There is some evidence that oxytocin plays a role in OCD, though how and when are not clear. Some adults with OCD have been found to have elevated **cerebrospinal fluid** levels of oxytocin. Some patients with Tourette syndrome who also had OCD had low levels of cerebrospinal fluid oxytocin.

Cerebrospinal fluid

Fluid that surrounds and fills the spaces within the brain and the spinal cord; also found in the spaces around nerve cells in the brain that neurotransmitters pass through.

Genetic Factors

Even though there are clear instances of family members having OCD, particularly parents and their children, studies of genetic linkage and of specific "candidate" genes that may be the cause have produced mixed and unclear results. This area is obviously of extreme interest, and it is likely that more clarity will develop in the coming years.

Environmental Factors

Although perhaps not a true "cause" of OCD, certain environmental factors can trigger the appearance of OCD or, in patients already suffering with OCD, can worsen some symptoms. Well-identified external factors include abuse of any kind, changes in living situation, other medical illness, death of a loved one, school-related problems, relationship problems, and other life stresses.

Psychological Theories

Before the modern era of medicine and the realization that biological factors can produce psychiatric disease, psychological theories were created to explain the cause of OCD .

Psychoanalytic theories: Freud classified OCD as a psychoneurosis. He said that the root of the illness is a disturbance in the sexual life or the development of the child who goes through the stages of oral, anal, and oedipal sexual interest. During or just before the oedipal phase, there may be a conflict between the **ego** (the "organized self") and the **id** (the "instinctive self"). The ego solves the conflict by trying to reduce the effect of the id, even if the solution is unpleasant. One compromise might be to regress to the previous phase of development (anal) and **hoard** (e.g., not want to throw anything away). Another compromise might be to act against an unconscious wish; for example, checking the oven might be interpreted as a way to deal with an aggressive wish to burn the house down. Today these formulations seem to have more to do with developmental difficulties, which would produce a personality disorder in adulthood and not OCD.

Cognitive theories: These theories suggest that obsessions represent catastrophic misinterpretations of an individual's thoughts, images, and impulses. Overestimation of threat, perfectionism, and intolerance of uncertainty are examples of faulty cognitive processes.

Streptococcal Infections

Some children develop OCD symptoms after streptococcal bacterial infections. This reaction to infection may be seen in 10% to 20% of children who develop OCD. It is an autoimmune disorder caused by the body producing an immune response (antibodies) to the streptococcal bacteria, which also seem

The Basics of OCD

Ego

The self, a conscious part of the mind.

Id

The unorganized part of the personality structure that contains the basic drives. The id is unconscious (as per Freud's original description).

Hoarding

The excess storing of food, money, or other goods.

Cognitive

Pertaining to cognition, the process of being aware, knowing, thinking, learning, and judging.

PANDAS

A diagnosis used to describe a set of children thought to have a rapid onset of OCD and/or tic disorders following group A beta-hemolytic streptococcal (GABHS) infections.

to attack the basal ganglia of the brain. In these patients, the symptoms usually start with tics. This condition is known as pediatric autoimmune neuropsychiatric disorders associated with streptococcal infections (**PANDAS**). A similar mechanism has been associated with kidney disease seen after streptococcal infection.

Neuropsychological Factors

Studies have shown that there are significant problems in visual-spatial integration in children with OCD. There may also be memory and reasoning problems.

PART TWO

The Diagnosis

What are the symptoms of OCD that I may see in my child?

Should I be concerned about my child's superstitions?

As a parent, what should I look for in our child? I don't want to miss seeing or doing something that will help our child.

More . . .

9. What are the symptoms of OCD that I may see in my child?

Children with OCD usually have both obsessions and compulsions but sometimes only one or the other. Attention is needed when symptoms persist, make no sense, cause significant distress, interfere with normal functioning (i.e., at school, with friends, or in relationships at home), or take up more than an hour a day. At this level, these symptoms are beyond "normal." (See Table 1.)

Obsessions are accompanied by uncomfortable feelings such as fear, disgust, doubt, or a belief that things have to be done "just right."

Obsessions

These are thoughts, images, or impulses that occur again and again and that seem to be out of control. The child does not want to have these ideas and finds them very disturbing and intrusive. The child usually knows that these are not realistic but cannot control them. Obsessions are accompanied by uncomfortable feelings such as fear, disgust, doubt, or a belief that things have to be done "just right."

Table 1   Common Types of Obsessions

Type	Associated Behaviors/Thoughts
Aggressive	Urge to stab someone or to push someone down
Morbid	Urge to harm oneself or others; thoughts of death and diseases
Religious	Blasphemous thoughts against God; thoughts of being possessed by the devil
Sexual	Thoughts of being homosexual; thoughts of having sex with an animal
Reviewing conversations	Urge to recall exactly what was said
Need to know	Intrusive questions that have no relevance to the current situation
Somatic	Excessive concern about being sick
Right and wrong	Obsession about having just the right thought before doing something
Obsession with light	Excessive focus on luminous objects

Compulsions

These are actions performed by the child to try to make the obsessions go away. Compulsions are acts that are performed over and over again according to certain rules or rituals. They do not give pleasure (contrary to compulsive drinking or gambling in adults, which often does give pleasure). These rituals are performed to obtain some relief from the discomfort (anxiety) caused by the obsessions (Table 1).

OCD symptoms usually change over time, sometimes being very minimal or sometimes producing extreme distress. They tend to wax and wane.

Some ritualistic behaviors and superstitions are normal during childhood development. However, the diagnosis of OCD becomes more likely with the following factors:

- Excessive frequency of obsessive-compulsive activities
- Excessive time spent on these activities
- Impaired functioning at home and in school
- Excessive level of anxiety
- Continuance of these behaviors past the time when they should disappear

OCD may worsen or cause disruptive behaviors, exaggerate a preexisting learning disorder, cause problems with attention and concentration, or interfere with learning in school.

Another way to look at OCD is to think of it as an "overactive system." The worry is so strong that a child feels that she or he must perform the task or dwell on the thought over and over again to the point where it interferes with everyday life. The child may realize that it is not necessary to repeat the behavior, but the anxiety is so high that he or she feels that the repetition is required to neutralize the painful feeling.

10. Does my daughter understand that this is not normal?

Insight

The ability to recognize one's own mental illness or mental state. An insight is the derivation of a rule that links cause with effect.

Most children with OCD recognize that the obsessions are coming from their own minds and are not realistic. They see that the compulsions they perform are excessive and unreasonable. Their **insight** is good in these cases. But some children do not have good insight and do not realize that their beliefs and actions are unreasonable.

Young children, in general, have poor insight about these problems and might not even be able to describe their symptoms well.

Young children, in general, have poor insight about these problems and might not even be able to describe their symptoms well. They may not have the cognitive capacity to understand the nature of the obsessions and of the compulsions, which may delay the diagnosis.

Another concern is oppositional children or older adolescents who may not want to admit there is something wrong with their behaviors. They may try to hide their actions and concerns, which can make diagnosis quite difficult.

11. My daughter is always worried about numbers. Is this unusual in OCD, and what other kinds of obsessions may she have in the future?

Many kinds of obsessions have been described. Common ones include:

- Contamination fears of germs, dirt, or environmental toxins
- Disgust with bodily wastes or secretions
- Fears that they are contaminated or that they may contaminate others
- Fears of having inadvertently harmed someone else
- Fear that something terrible may happen (e.g., fire, death, illness of a loved one, harm to self or others)
- Fear of losing control of aggressive urges

- Intrusive sexual thoughts, urges, or images
- Excessive religious or moral doubt
- "Forbidden" thoughts
- A need to have things "just so"
- A need to confess, to tell, or to ask something
- A need for symmetry, order, or exactness
- Concerns about lucky or unlucky numbers
- Preoccupation with sounds, words, or music
- Preoccupation with household items (e.g., toys, knives)

These are just some common examples. There are many others described by patients, and some may be influenced by the culture or environment of the child (e.g., cartoon characters, movies, celebrities).

One parent said:

We knew that our son Jonas was an anxious child, but it was only when he became an adult that we understood that he had suffered from OCD as a child. He only recently told us that when he was very young, maybe 7 years old, he was feeling overwhelmed and was afraid that bad things would happen. To prevent this, he felt the urgency to count everything. He also said that in the bathroom, he would spend a lot of time brushing his teeth because he would brush each tooth three times. He would wash his hands five times each. He would put his toiletry objects in a certain order before starting to wash. When watching television, he had to tap his feet on the floor, first his right foot two times and then his left foot two times. If he made a mistake in the order or the numbers, he had to do it all over again. Now, I remember that he had very dry hands even though I would buy all sorts of different moisturizing creams with little improvement, but I thought it was the weather or fragile skin. I never thought it could be due to excessive hand washing. I feel so guilty now. I didn't understand what he was struggling with at the time, and I didn't provide him with the medical help that could have made his life easier.

12. My son seems to wash his hands all the time. I guess this is a compulsion. What other kinds of compulsions might we see in him?

There are two broad groups of compulsions. The first is ideational compulsions, which involve mental conceptualization; the second is motor compulsions, which involve movement.

Ideational compulsions involve thinking processes. They include mental counting; using ritualized thought patterns, such as picturing specific things or repeating words or sentences; special prayers repeated in a set manner; mental list making; and mental reviewing. (See Table 2.)

Table 2 Common types of ideational compulsions

Type	Associated Behaviors
Counting	Mentally ordering objects, numbers, or words in some "favorable" combination
List making	Making mental lists of shopping items or activities
Praying	Praying mechanically without religious finality

Motor compulsions may be of four types:

- The aggressive type includes hair pulling, self-hitting, cutting, and head banging.
- The physiological type includes defecation, urination, eating, drinking, smoking, swallowing, or performing sexual acts.
- The movement type includes touching, tics, clapping, squeezing, jumping, stretching, throat clearing, rocking, rubbing, and exercising.
- The ceremonial type includes hand washing, showering, house cleaning, the need to ask or to confess, checking, arranging, checking repeatedly for signs of illness, retracing previous actions.

In addition to hand washing (i.e., the getting rid of dirt to the point where the hands become raw and inflamed), other compulsions commonly seen include:

- Showering or teeth brushing for very long periods of time
- Repeating the same action such as going in and out of doorways or up and down from a chair
- Needing to move through spaces in a special way (e.g., without touching anything, or covering one's hands with gloves or tissues)
- Checking multiple times to see if the house door is locked or the stove is turned off
- Examining completed homework many times to be sure it is done
- Touching the iron over and over to be sure it is cold
- Counting all the time to bring good luck
- Ordering or arranging objects in a certain manner, such as by numbers, by colors, or by size
- Hoarding or saving objects that are not necessary to keep
- Praying frequently to be forgiven for recurrent bad thoughts or saying the same prayer a certain amount of times
- Taking measures to prevent harm to oneself, such as locking away all household sharp objects
- Cleaning rituals in one's bedroom or elsewhere in the house and other similar repetitive actions

See Table 3 for more on compulsions.

13. How are obsessions and compulsions related? What do they have in common?

Obsessions and compulsions should not be viewed as separate entities. They have elements in common.

Both obsessions and compulsions intrude persistently and forcefully into the child's conscious awareness and produce a feeling of anxious dread. The symptoms are experienced as foreign to the child's experience of himself or herself. The child may or may not recognize that these obsessions and compulsions are absurd and irrational. This insight often depends on the developmental level of the child, with an older child more likely to understand the irrationality of the

Both obsessions and compulsions intrude persistently and forcefully into the child's conscious awareness and produce a feeling of anxious dread.

Table 3 Common Types of motor compulsions

Type	Associated Behaviors
Aggressive	Verbal or physical outbursts
Physiological	Spitting, defecating, swallowing
Movement	Touching, squeezing, throat clearing, rocking
Cleaning, washing	Long showers, handwashing, housecleaning
Checking	Locks, knobs, house appliances, written work
Repeating	Rewriting, rereading, redoing previous steps a few times
Counting	Counting out loud
Ordering, arranging	Organizing according to color, shape, size
Hoarding, collecting	Amassing magazines, shopping bags, mail
Need to ask, confess	Providing information not needed or seeking reassurance
Retracing	Getting out of bed the same way as getting into it
Somatic	Checking one's body for signs of illness

situation. There is usually a strong desire to resist the obsessions and compulsions. The symptoms are time consuming and may impair the child's functioning.

The symptoms are most frequently related in that the compulsion is done to relieve the anxiety produced by the obsession. For example, hand washing or taking a long shower will be done to try to reduce the fear of being dirty or contaminated; rereading homework many times may occur when the child is afraid that he or she may have written something inappropriate in it. Because the ritual temporarily reduces the anxiety, it is self-reinforcing.

Parents of 9-year-old Sarah said:

Our Sarah does not want to be touched (no handshaking or high fives for her). She refuses to sit on a couch with other people. She worries if she thinks she has brushed up against someone else.

She keeps her possessions in her room and does not let anyone use them (CDs, pens, clothes). She "panics" and has a temper tantrum if somebody uses a pen from her desk or sits on her bed—now the object has germs and she will get sick. Sometimes she asks me to wash her clothes again that just came out of the dryer if they were washed with other family members' clothes—they are dirty and she could catch a disease. So now I have to do a separate laundry load for her. She avoids touching things in public, and I have seen her turning door knobs after protecting her hand with her long sleeve or with a tissue. She washes after school.

14. Everybody worries sometimes. Why did the doctor say my child has a disease? What kinds of symptom patterns are we likely to see in our son that are so different from just worrying?

More than likely your doctor has determined that the extent of your child's thoughts, symptoms, and actions are excessive compared to the normal actions of another child of the same age and in the same circumstances. It can sometimes be hard to know if your child has crossed the "border" from normal thoughts and actions seen at that age into the area where OCD needs to be considered.

In some cases, the evidence from the child's behavior and actions is clear. In many other cases, though, the distinction from normal is not clear and the child may outgrow his or her behavior. The doctor may choose to watch and wait several months (with interval visits) to see if the behavior is at the "upper limit of normal" or if it moves into the OCD diagnosis. Like many other diseases, both medical and psychiatric, there is a continuum or spectrum of seriousness, with some people being barely ill and others quite severely. As the disease may evolve and change, the diagnosis may be unclear for a while.

OCD research is indicating a way of clustering symptom patterns by the patient's course, genetic risk, neuropathology, and treatment. At this point four models, or patterns, are described but there may be more. Note that a patient may show more than one pattern. Hence the percentages below may total more than 100%.

- The most common pattern is the obsession of contamination (45% in adults, 30% in children), accompanied by compulsive avoidance of the feared contaminator or by washing (50% in adults, 60% in children).
- The second is the need for symmetry or precision (31% in adults, 12% in children) with counting, arranging, ordering, and repeating compulsions. These patients take a very long time to achieve daily routine acts like eating or taking a shower.
- The third is the intrusion of sexual or aggressive thoughts (54% in adults but only 3% in children), religious thoughts, or somatic (body) obsessions, which include compulsions like checking or repeating a prayer multiple times. These children may feel compelled to report to the police or confess to a priest.
- The fourth is hoarding obsessions and collection compulsions. Studies have indicated that this subtype of OCD may have a different neurobiological mechanism.

Ron, a 17-year-old, said:

I have always been afraid of many things, like cheating during a test or lying or cursing at someone. Sometimes I get obsessed with bad racial thoughts. This is not me, as I have been raised in a very open-minded, religious family. I go to church regularly and believe in God. I do good things for others. However, in spite of that, bad thoughts pop up, and I fear that I will lose control and do something bad or hurt somebody else's feelings. It is so scary that I make myself walk 10 steps ahead and then turn around and walk 10 steps back. Counting and walking at the same time make me forget the bad thoughts. If I am with people, to avoid dealing with them, I tend to use a fake excuse, like saying I need to go and pick up a paper or an object.

15. Are there any rarer problems we might see?

Yes, you could encounter some other rare motor, **neurological**, and perceptual problems.

Neurological

Refers to functions controlled by the brain.

- Rare motor disturbances can include "freezing" behavior (lack of movement), involuntary movements, hyperkinesias (tremors or involuntary muscle contractions), tics, twitches, grimaces, tremors, and spasms.
- Neurological problems include abnormalities in fine motor coordination, involuntary movements, and mirror movements (i.e., the same movement occurring involuntarily on both sides of the body).
- Perceptual disturbances may also be observed, such as changes in smell and taste, visual disturbances, and compulsive staring into light bulbs or the sun, which may produce severe, sometimes permanent disease in the retina of the eye and blindness.

16. Is it possible that my child can become physically ill because of so much worrying?

Children with OCD frequently do not feel well and are prone to stress-related ailments such as headaches or upset stomachs (or irritable bowel syndrome). They are often tired due to a lack of sleep, as they are unable to fall asleep due to their worries or due to going to bed late after performing their rituals. These children are often referred to a mental health clinic by a pediatrician who recognizes the OCD symptoms, by a dermatologist who was consulted for irritated skin due to prolonged showers or frequent hand washing, or by a dentist consulted for gum problems related to the child's excessive brushing.

Children with OCD frequently do not feel well and are prone to stress-related ailments such as headaches or upset stomachs.

17. How do psychiatrists diagnose OCD?

Unlike many medical diseases that can be clearly diagnosed by blood tests, x-rays, or various other laboratory tests, OCD is diagnosed by a **psychiatrist** based on a combination of

Psychiatrist

A medical doctor (MD) specializing in the treatment of mental diseases and disorders. Psychiatrists are legally permitted to prescribe medications.

The Diagnosis

symptom descriptions, reported behaviors, observations, and secondary findings (e.g., irritated hands from excessive washing). Unfortunately there are no lab tests to make the diagnosis of OCD or most other mental health problems.

Following many years of study and experience, the American Psychiatric Association has defined the diagnosis criteria for OCD (and other mental health disorders) in a book called *Diagnostic and Statistical Manual of Mental Disorders*, which is now in its fourth edition with text revisions (**DSM-IV-TR**). This book covers the diagnosis of most psychiatric diseases and is the gold standard in psychiatry. Here are some of the criteria for OCD based on the *DSM-IV-TR*:

(DSM-IV-TR)

Reference textbook of classifications used by mental health professionals to diagnose people with mental disorders.

The child must have obsessions (recurrent and persistent thoughts, impulses or images) that are intrusive and cause distress, cannot be ignored and can be recognized as being created by the child or the child must have compulsions (repetitive behaviors or mental acts) performed as an effort to reduce the perceived anxiety. These symptoms occupy much of the child's time and have to interfere with daily activities. They cannot be the direct effect from the use of illicit drugs or medications. They cannot be due to a co-existing medical condition. The child may not recognize that his or her symptoms are abnormal and excessive (compared to adults who usually have more insight and can tell that they are having a problem).

Eva, a 15-year-old, said:

I feel so guilty when I argue with my brother or my mom. Sometimes, just looking at a friend the wrong way makes me sick. I always feel the need to apologize, and people get upset with me because they do not understand why I apologize so often. I would even go to confess to my priest if I could, even though I have been told that I am not sinning. Maybe this would make me feel better. I feel that nobody in my family understands me and that my friends try to avoid me. It makes me feel so lonely. Instead of apologizing, I try to recite numbers in my head or out loud if I am alone (doing it out loud is better because God hears me better and forgives me). If I start counting, I have to use only the "good numbers" like 1 or 3 or 7 and not "bad numbers" like 6 or 9 or 13. If I say the good numbers, it calms me. But if a bad number pops into my head, I have to start it all over.

18. What other mental problems are sometimes confused with OCD?

Some disorders share superficial similarities to OCD. They include:

Addictions: Adolescents with OCD may have substance abuse problems. Some adolescents may use alcohol or marijuana in order to not feel the distress related to the OCD. Pathological gambling is rare but may exist in adolescents, particularly through the Internet. Compulsive sexual activity is also seen. Compulsive masturbation is sometimes seen in developmentally delayed children.

Tic disorders: Tic disorders such as Tourette syndrome and other motor or vocal tic disorders may resemble OCD. Tics are involuntary motor or vocal behaviors that occur in response to a feeling of discomfort. Some complex tics, like touching or tapping, may resemble compulsions. Tics and OCD occur together more often when the OCD or the tics start in childhood.

Depression: Depression and OCD frequently occur together. Patients who have only depression rarely have the intrusive thoughts seen in OCD. People with OCD are usually not sad and can get pleasure from doing what they usually enjoy doing.

Post–traumatic stress disorder (PTSD): OCD can be made worse by stress. The differentiation can be made from PTSD because OCD is not caused by a dramatic event.

Depression

A state of lowered mood, usually with disturbances of sleep, appetite, suicidal thoughts, and so forth.

Post-traumatic Stress Disorder (PTSD)

An anxiety disorder that can develop after exposure to one or more terrifying events that threatened or caused grave physical harm.

Autism

A brain development disorder that impairs social interaction and communication; causes restricted and repetitive behavior, all starting before a child is 3 years old.

Asperger syndrome

One of several autism spectrum disorders (ASD) characterized by difficulties in social interaction and by restricted, stereotyped patterns of behavior, interests, and activities.

Schizophrenia

A psychiatric disorder characterized by psychosis with delusions and hallucinations.

Ego-dystonic

Behaviors that are in conflict with the ego—i.e., in conflict with a person's ideal self-image.

Ego-syntonic

Behaviors consistent with one's ideal self-image.

Developmental disorders: Children with pervasive developmental disorders, such as **autism** or **Asperger syndrome**, may have very stereotyped, rigid, compulsive behaviors, but they also have other severe difficulties with communication and with relating to other people (connecting) that do not exist in OCD.

Psychosis: **Schizophrenia**, delusional disorders, and other psychotic conditions may be differentiated because people with OCD understand quite well what is real and what is not.

19. What is obsessive-compulsive personality disorder? Is this different from OCD? Can my child have both?

Yes, obsessive-compulsive personality disorder (OCPD) is different from OCD. The two are often confused. OCPD is not diagnosed in children or adolescents less than 18 years of age because their personalities are still developing. However, certain features of this diagnosis (e.g., rigidity, perfectionism, stubbornness, preoccupation with rules and details) may already be present in children and may become clearer as they get older.

OCD is what is called **ego-dystonic**, meaning that the disorder is not compatible with the patient's self-concept (i.e., one's knowledge and understanding of who and what he or she is) and causes distress.

OCPD is **ego-syntonic**, meaning that the individual accepts his or her characteristics and "personality" and has no distress. People with this disorder are not aware of anything abnormal about themselves. They feel their actions are rational, and it is impossible to convince them otherwise. People with OCD are ridden with anxiety, while those with OCPD are not.

People with the personality disorder derive pleasure from their behaviors (e.g., they may enjoy their rigidity or their over-cleanliness). Treatment is usually by psychotherapy rather than medications. Freud was one of the first to describe this condition. He called it the anal-retentive character.

Your child cannot have OCPD, as this is diagnosed in adults only. OCD does not become OCPD. However, adults may have both.

20. Are there brain or neurological diseases that produce OCD symptoms? Could my child have a brain tumor or cancer?

There are some neurological diseases that could produce symptoms similar to OCD. These diseases include:

> *Tourette syndrome*: This syndrome is characterized by multiple tics (involuntary rapid movements or vocalizations). Individuals with Tourette syndrome may also have OCD and/or attention deficit hyperactivity disorder (ADHD). Up to 50% of people with Tourette syndrome also have OCD, but only a small percentage of children with OCD have Tourette syndrome. This disorder is often inherited. Relatives of individuals with Tourette syndrome may have OCD without the tics.

> *Encephalitis*: Encephalitis is an inflammation or infection of the brain, usually due to bacteria or viruses. Encephalitis can present with OCD symptoms.

> *Sydenham chorea*: This disease is characterized by rapid, uncoordinated, involuntary, non-repetitive, jerking movements affecting primarily the face, feet, and hands. It results from childhood infection with group-A beta-hemolytic streptococci.

Epilepsy and seizure disorders: Epilepsy is a recurrent seizure disorder caused by abnormal electrical discharges in the brain. It comprises a group of disorders for which recurrent seizures are the main symptom. The different forms of epilepsy are either secondary to a particular brain abnormality or neurological disorder, or are said to be "idiopathic," without any clear cause. Epilepsy can present with OCD symptoms.

ADHD: This disorder may also be due to neurological problems in addition to being considered a psychiatric problem. OCD is believed to share a genetic component with ADHD.

Brain injuries: Onset of obsessions and compulsions following a brain injury has been described in children.

Temporal lobe pathology: OCD symptoms have been seen in conjunction with **temporal lobe epilepsy**.

Basal ganglia disorders: The **basal ganglia** in the brain represents a processing area for information. It also controls voluntary movement, balance, and some reflexes. OCD symptoms have developed in older patients who had an infarction in their basal ganglia. A case was described of enlargement of the basal ganglia in an adolescent who had PANDAS and developed OCD symptoms.

These diagnoses are also complex and require the assistance of a neurologist and other medical tests (e.g., **electroencephalograms**, scans).

Brain tumors or cancers that present or begin with OCD-like symptoms are rather rare, and there are only a few reports of such cases in the medical literature. The likelihood of a tumor or cancer that presents with OCD symptoms is very low.

Temporal lobe epilepsy

Epilepsy in which epileptic origins are located in the temporal lobe of the brain. The temporal lobe is the lower section of the brain that controls memory and language comprehension.

Basal ganglia

Also referred to as the striatum. A group of interconnected nuclei that lies deep within the brain. Each of the nuclei (and its connections to other brain structures) appears to be involved in certain disorders, like ADHD, tics, Parkinson disease, and chorea.

Electroencephalogram (EEG)

A test that measures brain electrical activity and is particularly useful in looking for seizure disorders.

21. Do children with OCD experience delusions? And what is the difference between a delusion and an obsession? What is the difference between a delusion and an overvalued idea?

Delusions are rare in children, so they are generally not seen in children with OCD. A delusion is an unshakable belief in something untrue. The belief is not one ordinarily accepted by other members of the person's culture or subculture (e.g., it is not an article of religious faith). These irrational beliefs defy normal reasoning and remain firm even when overwhelming proof is presented to dispute the patient. Delusions are extremely fixed and impossible to change.

Delusion
A fixed, false belief.

Overvalued ideas are transient strong beliefs representing a false or exaggerated belief sustained beyond reason or logic but with less rigidity than a delusion. They are less unbelievable, and the patient may alter his or her idea somewhat with therapy.

An obsessive thought is a recurrent and persistent thought that is experienced as intrusive and inappropriate and that causes marked anxiety or distress.

22. Are there any other disorders that might be mistaken for OCD?

There are various conditions that have obsessive-compulsive qualities that are quite similar to OCD. These disorders are frequently described as obsessive-compulsive spectrum disorders (Table 4). They may even respond to some of the same treatments.

There is no clear consensus as to whether the relationship of these problems to OCD is deeper than just clinical similarities or whether they are **comorbid** with OCD.

Comorbid
When two disorders exist at the same time in the same individual.

Table 4 Obsessive Compulsive Spectrum Disorders

Psychiatric disorder	Other Terms for the Disorder	Characteristics	Comments
Trichotillomania	Compulsive hair pulling	Playing compulsively with and pulling hair	Usually only present with hair pulling without evolution to non-self-injurious compulsive rituals.
Body Dysmorphic disorder	Imagined ugliness; bodily shame; dysmorphophobia; body dysmorphia	Worrying constantly about one's appearance	32% of body dysmorphic patients experience OCD.
Stereotypic Movement Disorders	Previously called habit disorders	Thumb sucking, nail biting, nose picking, breath holding, bruxism (teeth grinding), head banging, rocking/rhythmic movements, self-biting, self-hitting, picking at the skin, hand shaking, hand waving, and mouthing of objects	The repetitive compulsive behaviors may superficially resemble OCD; frequently seen in severe development disorders like autism, Asperger syndrome, or mental retardation syndromes.
Eating Disorders	**Anorexia nervosa** or boulimia	Excessive focus on food and exercise	37% of anorexia nervosa patients have comorbidity with OCD. Individuals with **bulimia nervosa** have much lower rates of comorbidity with OCD (3%).
Hypochondria	Health anxiety; hypochondriasis	Obsessive, irrational fear of having a serious disease or medical condition	Classified in the somatoform disorders.
Compulsive skin picking		Repetitive picking at one's own skin, to the extent that it causes damage	23% of those with OCD may have compulsive skin picking.
Olfactory Reference Syndrome (ORS)	Autodysomophobia	Obsessive, irrational fear that one's body is emitting a foul, unpleasant odor; believing others' behaviors or comments are related to the imagined odor (e.g., someone else's cough, sneeze, or turning of the head is due to the alleged odor)	May be a subtype of OCD.

Children with OCD are at high risk to have other psychiatric disorders (Table 5). Most studies have found that up to 70% of children with OCD have at least one comorbid disorder. This comorbidity can make the diagnosis and treatment plan very complex and usually requires professional mental health intervention.

23. What is ritual play, and is it always abnormal? What is the difference between a normal child's ritual and that of a child with OCD?

Ritualistic play, superstitions, repetitive behaviors, and games are seen in all children at times during their development. There is actually a wide spectrum of ritualistic behaviors and actions, and it is only when obsessions and compulsions move to the extreme that they are considered to be signs of OCD. Rituals are used by children to master normal developmental anxieties and to help with socialization.

At about 2 years of age, it is common to see various bedtime rituals and the demand that things be "just so." The usual and familiar way is preferred at mealtimes, bathing, and bedtimes. Transitions are difficult, and there is often some anxiety about separation.

By 3 or 4 years of age, children become less rigid about their rituals and are more comfortable in dealing with change. For example, they may still be afraid of the dark and want the parent to stay with them longer by involving them in some sort of ritual before bed such as story reading or tucking in.

Normal contamination fears are seen at 6 to 11 years of age. For example, boys say that girls have "cooties," and they try to avoid touching them. By age 7, many children collect objects as a hobby. This collecting is different from hoarding (saving useless objects). As a hobby, kids collect objects meaningful to them and their peers. By age 8 or 9, children do not need the old rituals, and only occasional reassurance is necessary.

Most studies have found that up to 70% of children with OCD have at least one comorbid disorder.

Anorexia nervosa

An eating disorder characterized by low body weight and body image distortion with an obsessive fear of gaining weight.

Bulimia nervosa

An eating disorder in which patients are obsessed about weight, binge on food and then purge (vomiting or laxative use), or use excessive exercise to achieve their concept of thin.

The Diagnosis

Table 5   Psychiatric Disorders

Type of Disorder	Subtype	Comments
Anxiety disorders	Social phobia	11% comorbidity with OCD
	Simple phobia	7% comorbidity with OCD
	Panic disorders	6% comorbidity with OCD
	Generalized anxiety	Frequent in children with OCD
	Refusal to go to school	Frequent in children with OCD
	Separation anxiety	Frequent in children with OCD
Eating disorders	Anorexia Nervosa	More common in girls; more common in OCD patients than in the general population; OCD symptoms common in anorexia nervosa
Mood disorders	Bipolar disorder	If associated with OCD, OCD symptoms more serious and more difficult to treat; some medications might be problematic
	Depression	Frequently associated with OCD; OCD may cause the depression (i.e., patient not able to handle the symptoms of OCD) or coexistence
	Post-traumatic stress disorder (PTSD)	4% to 22% of people with PTSD have OCD symptoms; 54% of OCD patients had experienced at least one traumatic event in their lifetime
Somatoform disorder	Hypochondriasis; fear of AIDS	Fears of having a serious disease
Attention deficit disorders (ADHD, ADD)		In one study, 25% of children with OCD had associated ADHD
Learning disorders		OCD may worsen such a condition
Conduct disorders		OCD may worsen such a preexisting condition; however, in children with only OCD who have become disruptive, the treatment of the OCD may improve the behavior
Substance abuse		Risk is mildly increased in adolescents with OCD

Type of Disorder	Subtype	Comments
Pervasive developmental disorders	Autism; Asperger syndrome; childhood disintegrative disorder; **Rett syndrome**; pervasive developmental disorders not otherwise specified	Often exhibit stereotyped and repetitive motor mannerisms
Schizophrenia	Delusional disorders (rare in children)	OCD symptoms may exist

Ritualized play changes from being a solitary game to group play with rules in the games that have to be followed in a certain way by all the children.

During adolescence, it is common to see children becoming "obsessed" with a movie star, collecting the person's pictures, or spending days playing a favorite game related to this person. It is just a focused interest and often a fad that many of their peers have adopted too.

OCD rituals represent an excess of these normal developmental rituals or may take on a wholly different quality. OCD rituals have a later age of onset and are distressing if not performed. They interfere with the child's life and are excessive (checking, washing, and counting).

In OCD, unlike with normal rituals, indecisiveness and doubt can prevent the child from completing the tasks. Obstinacy may cause unwanted arguments with other children.

Rigidity makes the child unable to easily switch from one task to another as other children do.

Magical thinking, also called "thought–action fusion," may be seen in OCD and refers to the belief that if the child thinks something, it will occur. Sometimes this thinking may almost look delusional, and the child may be misdiagnosed as psychotic.

The Diagnosis

Conduct disorder
Disorder in which there is an active transgression of societal rules.

Rett syndrome
An inherited, X-linked neurological disorder that is fatal to males. In females, there is rapid neurological deterioration leading to dementia, autism, and loss of speech and voluntary movements.

Magical thinking
Refers to the belief that if the child thinks something, it will occur.

A child with OCD may be very controlling, and this need to be in charge can be problematic for family members or even for the therapist, as the child may be oppositional and refuse to do the homework given by the therapist.

Parent of 10-year-old Brian said:

What an ordeal for him to go to bed! Brian needs to look under his bed, to fluff his pillows in a certain way—from top to bottom only. He opens and closes his bedroom door twice to make sure it's closed. He goes to the bathroom again to check and see if the faucets are turned off. He makes sure that the front door is closed and locked 4 times. He turns the light on and off a few times to be sure it's off. He looks out of the window to be sure nobody is outside. He checks and rechecks until he feels that everything is just right. Sometimes it takes close to one hour to do this. If he does not do this, he cannot fall asleep. This is becoming ridiculous, and I get frustrated with him.

24. Should I be concerned about my child's superstitions?

No, most children go through a normal phase in which they act in "superstitious" ways. A superstition is a belief or notion not based on reason or knowledge. It could be an unreasonable or excessive belief in fear or magic. For example, children may not want to walk under a ladder for fear of bad luck or may hold their breath until they cross the street, which will help them succeed during a test at school. This behavior should not be confused with OCD. When children are in this phase, these beliefs are playful and are not really serious. Children can laugh about them and tell them to other kids. Also, they tend to disappear within weeks or months. In OCD, the fears or rituals are serious to the child and may not disappear very quickly. Because they are shameful, they are not told to others.

Superstition and magical beliefs are very common in the child and adult population as a whole. Many people still avoid walking under ladders or are mildly upset when a black cat crosses their path. There are still skyscrapers built "without" a 13th floor!

It is normal that a young child's thought processes include magical thinking and a belief that magic is real. This is why stories like *Harry Potter* resonate so well with children (and adults). Children between 6 and 8 years old may cross their fingers to protect themselves from telling a lie or may not walk on the cracks in the concrete sidewalk to prevent bad luck. In normal development, superstitious rituals tend to fade by 8 years of age. Stress and performance anxiety may produce superstitious behaviors in adolescents and even in adults (e.g., carrying a lucky charm).

In OCD, these beliefs cross a line and become excessive. Rather than decreasing anxiety, the superstitions may now increase anxiety. They become emotionally draining, wasting a lot of time and producing no evident benefit.

Although the abnormal thoughts and behaviors in OCD have some similarities to "normal" superstitions, they are more intense and they come from nowhere. Thus they are qualitatively and quantitatively different.

25. Could some of the symptoms be so bad or difficult that they will prevent my daughter from receiving benefit from treatment?

Yes, if your daughter is extremely frightened and distressed by her obsessions, she might be too preoccupied to relax enough to get involved in her treatment, in particular, the cognitive-behavioral therapy (see Question 46). She may need to be started first on medication to relieve the anxiety and to improve her sleep. If there is any associated depression, this will need to be addressed quickly as well. It will only be in a second treatment phase that the work on the obsessions and the compulsions can be done.

Although the abnormal thoughts and behaviors in OCD have some similarities to "normal" superstitions, they are more intense and they come from nowhere.

26. Will my son attack me or someone else? What is the risk of violence in OCD?

Intrusive thoughts may involve violent obsessions about hurting others or oneself. Thoughts of inflicting harm, such as jumping from a bridge, jumping in front of a train, or pushing another person in front of a car, are not uncommon. Patients also describe imagining or wishing harm to a family member or impulses to shout something violent. Children may worry that they will act on these thoughts and might ask their parents to lock away the house knives, or they may refuse to leave the house.

Fortunately, the possibility of acting upon these impulses is low because children with OCD are tormented by their symptoms and feel guilt and shame. There is danger only if children have additional feelings or symptoms such as intrusive violent thoughts that are not upsetting to them or are even pleasurable. These feelings are signs that violence might be possible. In addition, violence is a possible concern if the child has acted previously in a violent manner or hears voices saying to be violent, or if the child is psychotic or feels uncontrollable and irresistible anger. If any of these occur, professional help should be obtained immediately.

27. Is there a risk for suicide? What should I look for, and what should I do?

The risk for self-injury or suicide must also be assessed, particularly when there is an associated depression. OCD and depression may coexist in children. Children do try to kill themselves. However, they frequently do not understand what is needed to die. For example, a young child may swallow two vitamins in an attempt to commit suicide, and the family may not consider this a suicide attempt.

Young children cannot understand that death is irreversible and may think they will be able to come back to life later.

Young children cannot understand that death is irreversible and may think they will be able to come back to life later. Children sometimes make threats when angry that they do not mean. However, accidents happen. Be aware if your child is sad, is not sleeping well, has a poor appetite, is being more withdrawn, or is making statements like "I wish I was not here," "I wish I could die," "I don't like my life," "I don't like myself," or "Nobody likes me." Go immediately to a place where your child can be evaluated by a child psychiatrist. If your child is already in treatment and is receiving medications, contact the doctor immediately to discuss the issue and to see if this suicidal behavior might be an adverse effect of the medicine or if something else is going on. Do not wait for the next appointment. Risk for suicide is an emergency.

28. I read somewhere that infections can actually cause OCD. Is this true? What is PANDAS?

OCD is not an actual infection. There are no bacteria or viruses in the brain that cause OCD and that could be treated with antibiotics or anti-viral medications. However, there are a group of diseases sometimes seen after treated infections (bacterial and viral). OCD occurring after infection is known as PANDAS (pediatric autoimmune neuropsychiatric disorders associated with streptococcal infections).

The idea that some cases of OCD may be due to a previous infection is inspired by the disease model of another neuropsychiatric problem, Sydenham chorea, which in some cases may be seen after bacterial infections. Sydenham chorea is a neurological disease seen in patients who have previously been infected by certain types of group-A beta-hemolytic streptococci bacteria. It may occur as late as 6 months after the infection and may present with abnormal involuntary movements of the arms and legs as well as facial grimaces, weak muscle tone, loss of fine motor control, and trouble walking. This disease is usually seen in children younger than 18 years of age and is more frequent in girls. The problem may disappear in a few months but occasionally persists for years. A similar disease process could explain some cases of OCD that follow certain strep infections.

PANDAS is a group of disorders that includes OCD, Tourette syndrome, and other tic disorders that occur after certain streptococcal ("strep") infections (e.g., sore throat). Not all children with strep infections develop PANDAS or other post-infection diseases such as rheumatic fever. After the infection (even if successfully treated), in some children, OCD symptoms may occur. Sometimes the new onset of symptoms is abrupt and dramatic. Sometimes preexisting OCD symptoms become worse.

PANDAS is believed to be caused by the body's response to the bacteria. Antibodies are produced by the body as a normal response to an infection. However, in the case of PANDAS, the antibodies may attack not just the strep bacteria but also parts of the body such as the heart (in rheumatic fever) or the basal ganglia in the brain, producing or worsening OCD, Tourette syndrome, or other psychiatric/neurological problems. However, this theory is not yet proven. And even if this theory is true, it is not clear why this effect would occur in one child and not in another.

PANDAS is similar to Sydenham chorea but usually presents in a much shorter time after the infection and has fewer of the movement problems and more of the tics and the psychiatric manifestations, such as obsessions and compulsions identical to those in OCD. These OCD symptoms may begin 2 to 4 weeks before the onset of the abnormal movements.

There are five criteria needed for the diagnosis of PANDAS:

Chorea

Rapid, jerky, involuntary, irregular muscle movements or twitching.

- Presence of OCD and/or a tic disorder
- Onset before puberty
- An episodic course characterized by acute, severe onset and dramatic symptom exacerbations
- Neurological abnormalities such as **chorea**
- A clear temporal relationship between the strep infection and the symptoms

PANDAS exacerbations are typically quite dramatic. Patients report that the symptoms "came on overnight" or "appeared all of a sudden" a few days after a sore throat.

The major distinguishing feature of PANDAS patients is the history of the strep infection, which is not seen in classic OCD patients. Sometimes it is hard to make the diagnosis of the group-A beta-hemolytic streptococci infection, and throat cultures or blood anti-streptococcal **antibody** testing may be needed.

Of course, just because a child has strep throat does not mean he or she will also have PANDAS. Most school children have strep throat at some point, and the vast majority recover with no complications. Most children who have OCD or tics do not have PANDAS. The condition should be considered only if the OCD symptoms or tics are clearly, directly preceded by or significantly worsened after a strep infection.

29. How is PANDAS treated? Is it really OCD, and do you treat it the same way?

PANDAS is treated largely as classic OCD (see Part Three on treatment). Antibiotics are usually not required unless the child still has a strep infection. Two special treatment considerations are described here.

Plasmapheresis

One experimental method of treatment for PANDAS-related OCD is plasmapheresis, which is filtering of the child's blood to remove streptococcal antibodies. It is a difficult inpatient procedure requiring a few days' stay in the hospital. There are no significant studies reported for this treatment and only case reports of success. There is a high **incidence** of side effects, and it is not clear that this method is superior to other treatments. Nor is it clear whether the effects are long lasting. It should still be considered experimental and should not be a first choice of treatment in PANDAS.

Antibody

One of many proteins found on a particular type of white blood cell (B cell); is secreted into the blood or elsewhere after a stimulus (e.g., presence of bacteria).

Incidence

The number of cases or events per time period (for example, 100 new cases of infection per year in a town).

IVIG (Intravenous Immunoglobulin) Therapy

IVIG therapy involves an injection of a product made from pooled human blood donations approved by the **Food and Drug Administration (FDA)** for use in the treatment of various immunodeficiency and autoimmune diseases. In a small study of patients with PANDAS-related OCD, the effectiveness of this treatment appeared to be excellent. This relatively safe procedure can be done in an outpatient setting but is not approved by the FDA for this use. It is still considered experimental. The serious drawback to this treatment is its cost and the fact that many insurance companies have not covered it until now.

30. As a parent, what should I look for in our child? I don't want to miss seeing or doing something that will help our child.

Recognizing OCD is often difficult because the child becomes adept at hiding the questionable behaviors. It is not uncommon for a child to engage in ritualistic behavior for months or even years before parents know about it. The parents may think that the odd behavior is just a phase. Even though the child's behavior often takes up a great deal of time and energy, making it difficult to complete tasks such as homework or chores, he or she will still try to hide it due to shame or guilt. The child may compensate by sleeping less or skipping some activities or outings in order to complete the ritual. There may be serious problems with concentration because of the intrusive thoughts and lack of sleep.

In addition to feeling frustrated or guilty for not being able to control his or her own thoughts or actions, the child with OCD may have low self-esteem in comparing himself or herself to peers.

It is common at some point for the child to ask his or her parents to join in the ritualistic behavior and to seek frequent reassurance. In the beginning, parents may not realize that these are indications of OCD. If parents do not participate in the rituals, tantrums and difficult behaviors arise. The

It is not uncommon for a child to engage in ritualistic behavior for months or even years before parents know about it.

phenomenon in which family members participate in or facilitate a child's rituals is called family accommodation. It occurs in approximately 89% of OCD cases and is associated with dysfunctional family interactions, family distress, and greater OCD symptom severity. It was found also that the presence of comorbid oppositional defiant disorder (ODD) and family accommodation was a significant predictor of poor outcomes.

Parents should look for these possible signs of OCD:

- Raw, chapped hands from constant washing
- High rate of soap or paper towel usage
- High unexplained water bills (due to long showers)
- Unproductive hours spent apparently doing homework
- Holes in school test papers and homework due to writing and erasing words multiple times
- Requests for family members to repeat strange phrases
- A persistent fear of illness
- A sudden increase in laundry due to the child asking to clean the same clothes repeatedly
- Fear of germs
- A very long time spent getting ready to go to bed
- A permanent fear that something terrible will happen
- Constant checking of family members' health
- Reluctance to leave the house at the same time as other family members in order to perform rituals unnoticed

For more indications of OCD, see Questions 9, 11, and 12.

31. Is OCD due to bad parenting? What should we expect as parents of a child with OCD?

Absolutely not. The causes of OCD are external to the child's parents and caregivers.

When a child has OCD, the whole family is affected. Parents become confused and bewildered. This confusion sometimes comes across as frustration and anger. Children sometimes have episodes in which they are extremely angry with their parents, particularly if the parents do not allow or are unable to comply with the OCD demands and behavior (such as preventing the child from showering for hours at a time or refusing to wash the child's clothes multiple times). If parents overreact and attempt to interrupt the behaviors, the child may become hostile or extremely anxious. If parents give in to the rituals, the child never learns to confront his or her fears. Younger children who have a hard time articulating their needs may appear naughty, oppositional, "needy," or anxious and may have long and frequent temper tantrums.

Parents may be blamed by other family members for being too lenient toward the child (if they go along with the rituals) or being too strict and not understanding (if they refuse). The mother and father may have a different understanding of the situation and of the attitude to take. This disagreement often produces tension in the couple. A clever child may then play one parent against the other for his or her own advantage.

Having a child with a chronic illness is difficult to handle, and you will need all the support you can get—both familial and professional—to achieve positive results. The parents need to be united in order to be firm, supportive, and consistent in their rules for the child and in deciding upon the child's treatment course.

32. My son with OCD seems to act up only at home and never at school. How can this happen? If he can control himself there, why can't he do it at home?

This is common. Many children with OCD may be successful academically and with other school activities, but they may have difficulty completing their homework and papers, as they focus on getting things perfect. Many children, feeling embarrassed by their symptoms, successfully hide them from their peers and teachers but cannot hide them at home when they are more tired and less in control of their behaviors. They also know that they will not be judged in the same negative manner at home.

Many children, feeling embarrassed by their symptoms, successfully hide them from their peers and teachers but cannot hide them at home when they are more tired and less in control of their behaviors.

Your son should be evaluated for this problem because it is not clear that he will be able to continue to "hide" his symptoms while at school. The inevitable changes that occur at school (e.g., starting in a new school or grade, meeting new children, having more academic pressure) may cause the symptoms to appear in school at a more stressful time.

33. Are there any tests for OCD? Like brain scans or blood tests?

Unfortunately, there are no standardized tests that can be used to diagnose and track the treatment and progress of OCD. This is true for most psychiatric diseases. There are, as of yet, no blood tests, brain scans, or other such indicators that are routinely used in disease management.

Various structured tests have been developed to aid in diagnosing and assessing the severity of pediatric OCD and other anxiety disorders. They are primarily used in research studies rather than in standard clinical practice. These tests include:

- The Multidimensional Anxiety Scale for Children (MASC)—a test used for the assessment of anxiety in 8- to 19-year-olds. The test takes 1 to 2 hours to administer and provides an overall severity score, as well as descriptions and other scores that can help to classify the nature of the anxiety disorder.
- The Yale-Brown Obsessive Compulsive Scale (Y-BOCS)—the most frequently used scale. It is primarily used to assess adults and adolescents. It includes a symptom checklist and a severity rating. The range of severity for patients who have both obsessions and compulsions is: 0–7 **subclinical**; 8–15 mild; 16–23 moderate; 24–31 severe; 32–40 extreme. The severity rating scale may be used to monitor progress.
- The Children's Yale-Brown Obsessive Compulsive Scale (CY-BOCS)—a scale similar to the Y-BOCS. It is designed to establish the diagnosis of OCD in children by assessing current and past obsessions and

Subclinical

A condition or disease that shows no signs or symptoms and is detectable only by special tests.

compulsions. It rates the amount of time occupied by symptoms, the degree to which symptoms interfere in daily life, the amount of distress experienced, the internal resistance to doing the compulsion, and the control the child has over both obsessions and compulsions. This scale includes over 70 typical obsessions and compulsions. The severity scale also provides a way to assess and monitor the child's progress during treatment. A decrease of 25% or more is clinically significant.

- The Leyton Obsessional Inventory-Child Version (LOI-CV)—another widely used rating scale. It measures 20 items.
- A Family Accommodation Scale (FAS)—can be given to a family member to evaluate the family involvement in the child's symptoms.

As noted, these tests would not normally be used by your child's doctor during diagnosis or treatment unless you are in a medical research center where studies are underway.

Parents of 5-year-old Juan said:

Juan is always putting things in a certain order. Toys are placed in a certain way. When he takes his little car collection, he places the garbage truck first. Then, he places the police car next to it. Then comes the ambulance and then the bus. He does not play with them; he just places them in the same order again and again. If you change the order, Juan has a fit. And if you change the order with one of them sticking out a little bit, he gets upset and has to redo everything. Also, he will refuse to eat if the food is not placed in a symmetric way or unless different foods are aligned in a certain way. For example, at breakfast Cheerios are piled in each side of the bowl before milk can be poured into the center of the bowl between the two piles. Only then will Juan eat. Before going to bed, he puts his two pillows next to each other with the pillowcase openings facing each other, and then he puts a toy on each side of his pillows. He may have OCD. . .

PART THREE

The Treatment— General Concepts

What kinds of treatment choices do we have for our daughter's OCD?

Is there anything I can do to help in the treatment of my son's OCD?

How often should my son see the doctor?

More . . .

34. This has been a very difficult time with our son who appears to have OCD. My husband and I feel he needs to be seen and treated. Where do we go? What do we do now?

Most parents are concerned about their child's emotional health or their behavior, but they do not know where to find help. You can start by talking to friends, family members, your spiritual counselor, your child's school counselor, your child's pediatrician, or a family physician. Be cautious about using Yellow Pages phone directories as the only source of information or referral. Other sources may include:

- The employee assistance program through your employer
- The local medical or psychiatric society
- The local mental health association
- The town or county mental health department
- A local hospital with psychiatric services
- The Department of Psychiatry in a nearby medical school
- National advocacy organizations, such as National Alliance on Mental Illness (NAMI) National Mental Health Association (NMHA), or Federation of Families for Children's Mental Health
- National professional organizations, such as American Academy of Child and Adolescent Psychiatry (AACAP) or American Psychiatric Association (APA)

See the appendix for Web sites and contact information.

35. We went to a medical center for treatment, and they have psychiatrists, psychologists, psychiatric social workers, therapists, and lots of other kinds of mental health professionals. This is very confusing. What is the difference between all of them and whom should we see first?

Here is a brief description of the various professionals you may encounter in seeking help for your child:

- Child and adolescent psychiatrist—a licensed physician (MD or DO) who has trained for at least 3 years as a general (adult) psychiatrist after graduating medical school and who has 2 additional years of advanced training beyond general psychiatry with children, adolescents, and families. All child psychiatrists must first train as general psychiatrists.

  There are two rigorous national exams given by the American Board of Psychiatry and Neurology. The first is in general psychiatry and can be taken after completing general psychiatric training. The second is in child and adolescent psychiatry and can be taken after training in this area. Although passing the tests is not obligatory to practice psychiatry, many psychiatrists take these tests to demonstrate their mastery of the field. When a psychiatrist passes "the boards," he or she is said to be "board certified" in general psychiatry (the first exam) or in child and adolescent psychiatry (the second exam). A psychiatrist may be board certified in one or both areas. Someone who is "board eligible" has completed the required training after medical school and either has not taken the boards yet or has not passed them.

  Child and adolescent psychiatrists provide medical and psychiatric evaluation and a full range of treatment interventions for emotional and behavioral problems and psychiatric disorders. They may prescribe and monitor medications. They must be licensed by the state or province in which they practice.

- General or adult psychiatrist—a physician who has a medical degree (MD or DO) and at least 3 additional years of training primarily in adults. They may prescribe and monitor medications and must be licensed in their state or province. As noted previously, they may or may not be board certified.

- (Clinical) Psychologist—a person who has studied clinical psychology and has an advanced degree either at the master's level (MS) or the doctoral level (PhD, PsyD, or EdD) in clinical, educational, counseling, or research psychology. They are not physicians. Psychologists are licensed by their state. They can provide psychological evaluation and treatment for emotional and behavioral problems, psychological testing, and assessments. In most jurisdictions, they are not permitted to prescribe medications, as they are not physicians.

- Social worker—another professional who may play a role in treating patients with OCD. Some social workers have a bachelor's degree (BA, BSW, or BS). Many also have earned a master's degree (MS or MSW) or doctorate (PhD). They may take an examination to be licensed as clinical social workers and provide various forms of therapy. They do not prescribe medications, as they are not physicians.

You should ask prospective healthcare professionals whether they have experience treating OCD and, in particular, treating OCD in children.

You should find mental health professionals who are trained to work with children, adolescents, and families and particularly with experience in working with OCD patients. It is very important to find a good match between your child, your family, and the mental health professional because treatment and support may be needed for long periods of time.

You should ask prospective healthcare professionals whether they have experience treating OCD and, in particular, treating OCD in children. You may also want to understand how they approach OCD in terms of diagnosis and treatment.

Whom you see first will depend on what resources are available in your area. Usually, if you go to a local psychiatric clinic or center, an intake will be done first by a social worker. Then, the case will be discussed with other staff members, looking at the severity of the problem, before a referral is made for a psychiatric evaluation.

If you go privately for a consultation, it is a good idea to go first for a full evaluation by a child psychiatrist. A child psychiatrist can evaluate your child's full physical and emotional health, both as a developing individual and also in his or her familial and social context. Then, the child psychiatrist will help you coordinate all needed services and will follow your child regularly to evaluate the progression of the treatment. The psychiatrist is also the one who should monitor any psychiatric medications your child may be taking.

There are many different models you can follow with treatment teams (which are very common now) rather than assigning your child's care to a single individual. Teams may include social workers, psychologists, and child psychiatrists. It is generally not recommended that treatment of a child with OCD be done by a general (adult) psychiatrist or a team without experience treating OCD in children.

36. My daughter does not have a clear diagnosis of OCD. Rather it might be another mental problem or even OCD plus another problem? Do we treat both potential problems together or one after the other? If we treat one, will it make the other worse?

This case is clearly more complex than a simple and straightforward diagnosis of OCD in your child. In this situation, you should first be sure the treating psychiatrist has made all the appropriate efforts to clarify the diagnosis and then discuss with the doctor what the treatment plan is.

Keep in mind that the diagnosis may be very hard to establish in some cases. As your daughter develops, symptoms may become clearer and it may be easier to make the diagnosis definitively. Nonetheless, her child psychiatrist will be able to develop a treatment plan even if the diagnosis is not yet completely established.

As with all treatments in medicine and psychiatry, flexibility is needed in the treatment plan. If the initial plan is working well, it should be continued, but if it proves ineffective, you should discuss alternative treatments with the healthcare providers.

37. What kind of treatment choices do we have for our daughter's OCD ?

The first step in treating OCD is educating your daughter and the rest of your family about the disease and its treatment as a medical illness.

There are three components to the treatment of OCD in your daughter:

1. Education of the child and family: Education is crucial because it will help children and families learn how best to manage OCD and will help prevent its complications.
2. Psychotherapy: Cognitive-behavioral therapy (CBT) is the key element for most children and adolescents with OCD (See Question 46).
3. Medication: Medication using a serotonin reuptake inhibitor is helpful for many patients.

These three components of treatment will generally play out in two stages:

1. Acute treatment: This stage is aimed at ending the current episode of OCD.
2. Maintenance (relapse prevention) treatment: This stage is aimed at preventing future episodes of OCD.

Both stages clearly require teamwork involving the child, the family, and the treatment team.

38. Is there anything I can do to help in the treatment of my child's OCD?

First, you need to become an expert on the illness. Read books, study some of the online resources cited in the appendix of this book, attend lectures about OCD, talk with the therapist and the doctor. Join the Obsessive Compulsive Foundation (http://www.ocfoundation.org). Gather the support of your family or close ones and educate them about the illness.

You will, of course, need to do the usual things required in any medical treatment, such as getting your child to his or her appointments, ensuring the medication is taken (if prescribed), and being supportive and patient. Your monitoring of the symptoms is very valuable. Since you are usually with your child more than anyone else, you are one of the key individuals to help your child control and hopefully recover from his or her illness.

39. I assume the first visit to the psychiatrist will be important and may take a lot of time. What will the doctor do with my child on that first visit?

Initially there will be a comprehensive psychiatric evaluation. This evaluation usually requires several hours over one or more office visits for the child and the parents. With the parents' permission, other significant people (such as the child's pediatrician, school personnel, or other relatives) may be contacted for additional information.

The evaluation frequently includes the following:

- Description of the present problems and symptoms
- Information about health, allergies, surgery, and other illnesses and treatments (both physical and psychiatric), including past and current medications

- Parents' and family members' health and psychiatric histories to see if there is any genetic or familial component
- Child developmental history
- Information about school history and school performance
- Information about friends and hobbies
- Information about family relationships
- Psychiatric interview of the child
- If needed, special assessments such as psychological, educational, speech and language evaluations, neurological evaluations, or x-rays
- If medications are considered, blood tests and an **electrocardiogram (EKG)**

Electrocardiogram (EKG)

An electrical record of the heart that shows the heart's electrical currents; useful test to diagnose certain cardiovascular problems or disease.

The psychiatrist is there to be a partner to support your child and family, and to help, not to blame or judge. There is no guilt or fault to be assigned.

Then, the child psychiatrist will develop a report describing the child's condition and explain it to you in terms that you and your child understand. This report will include the biological, psychological, and social parts of the condition. The developmental needs, weaknesses, and strengths of your child will be included as well. Time will be given to answer questions.

The psychiatrist is there to be a partner to support your child and family, and to help, not to blame or judge. There is no guilt or fault to be assigned. You and your child do not need to worry about how you will be viewed during the evaluation. The psychiatrist will listen to your concerns and help to define a goal to achieve. You and your child should always ask questions if something covered is unclear.

The psychiatrist will offer treatment recommendations and describe benefits and risks of the recommended treatment so you and your child can feel comfortable with your decisions. A specific treatment plan is then developed, discussed, and accepted. Remember that flexibility is the key word here. Treatments will be modified until the best approach is found. In addition, as your child develops and grows up, the treatment that worked at 8 years of age may not work at age 10 or 12 and will need to be altered. You should expect and understand that changes will occur.

40. How often should my son see the doctor?

Visits will be fairly frequent at the beginning of the treatment. If your son is taking medications, it is likely that he will have blood tests and a physical examination (if he has not had one for a long time or if there is another medical problem). The doctor may want to increase the dosage of the medications and will want to make sure that it is well tolerated. Assessing any side effects will be done continuously, and changing dose or medication will be done as needed to get the best treatment effect.

Once your son is doing well, the appointments will be spaced out. A three visits per year schedule is common if your child is stable.

You will need to contact the doctor regardless of the appointment schedule if there is a worsening of the OCD symptoms, if there are side effects to the medication, if new symptoms appear such as depression or different kinds of anxieties (like **panic attacks** or **generalized anxiety** or phobias), or if any sort of crisis or stress occurs that worsens his OCD.

You should try not to miss appointments, as this may slow the progress or even allow your son to regress or become worse. It is harder to get OCD under control than to keep it controlled. To put it another way, it is harder to treat an acute worsening than to keep maintenance going. So do not risk a relapse by stopping or altering your son's treatment on your own. All treatment changes should be discussed with the psychiatrist. This adherence is particularly important because once the acute episode is over, your son will be on a maintenance (relapse-prevention) program. Changes to this program may increase the risk of a relapse.

Panic attack

A sudden, discrete period of intense anxiety, with physiological arousal.

Generalized anxiety disorder (GAD)

A constant, excessive worry with restlessness, fatigue, irritability, and sleep disturbances; GAD patients can also experience their minds going blank, muscle tension, and feeling on edge.

41. Can we take a vacation? We really need one. Will this harm our child? Will we miss therapy or treatment?

Of course you can take a vacation. If your child is stable and the doctor visits are every couple of months or so, indeed you should take a vacation. You should discuss the vacation with your child's physician and explain it clearly to your child in advance to calm his or her anxieties.

In the acute phase, however, if your child is not yet stable on treatment or is in a relapse, you may want to discuss with your physician the best way to handle such a trip.

42. Should I get a second opinion from another psychiatrist?

It depends. If you are satisfied with the treatment team you have, and if they are experienced and confident in their approach to your child's problem, then this should be sufficient—particularly if you see progress in the treatment and in your child's behavior.

But if you have any doubts or issues, or if the case is particularly complex, you may want to consider another opinion. In this case, it may be wise to head to a larger academic medical school or tertiary center that has strong child and adolescent psychiatry services. As always, this decision is very individual and personal.

If you have decided to get a second opinion, it is usually a good idea to discuss this with your child's psychiatrist. Although this matter may be delicate, a good and thorough psychiatrist will welcome a second opinion to "validate" his or her conclusions and to possibly add additional insight and experience. Your child's psychiatrist may even be able to recommend someone at his or her medical school or a professor or mentor.

43. *What is the role of family members in the treatment?*

Family members want to help their loved one. They will be willing to get educated about the disorder and to understand its causes and treatment. In some cases, family members may bring you new information (e.g., other cases in the family). They will help you cope with your child's symptoms. You may also find that they will help you communicate better with your child's therapist if it is difficult for you—they will be able to work as a team to support you.

Family members may be able to report to your child's therapist (with your consent) any symptoms that you might have over-looked or that do not occur in your presence. They may also help you by relieving you of certain tasks occasionally, such as helping with your child's homework or with the other children. Obviously, you must use discretion if you have certain family members who are not sympathetic or willing to help.

There are several things you should tell your family members:

- Understand that OCD is a disease and that your child is not responsible for all the symptoms. Ask family members not to criticize or make negative comments but rather to be calm and supportive. Let them know that even if they try to be helpful, your child may not be willing to receive their help. They must try to be kind and patient and not take any of your child's comments personally.
- Do not tell your child to stop the compulsive behavior, as it might make him or her feel worse; rather, use praise when seeing that your child is making an attempt to stop the behavior. Manage expectations—avoid expecting too much or too little, and do not push too hard.
- Focus on the positive. Learn treatment techniques from the therapist. Family members can try to follow the

child's homework so they can help if the child allows it. But remember that an adolescent may not be willing to be coached. Be alert to problems possibly due to the treatment. Do not attribute everything that goes wrong to OCD; a bad day might be just a bad day.

- Treat your child normally when he or she recovers. Be alert to any sign of relapse. Encourage the child to stick with the treatment, and be honest and open with the therapist.
- Family members may visit the therapist with your child if there is something they want to share or report.
- Family members should set consistent limits and let your child know what is expected. They should not be too lenient because your child has an illness.

Work with the school and the teachers as necessary. Do not hesitate to think about support groups for families. Take time for yourself to get refreshed so that you can better provide support later on.

44. What do I do if my daughter wants to stop taking her medications or stop seeing the doctor?

If your daughter feels like stopping the treatment, discuss this with her doctor. Do not stop or adjust the medications on your own.

If your daughter feels like stopping the treatment, discuss this with her doctor. Try to find out why. Is it side effects with medication or perhaps other kids teasing her? Do not stop or adjust the medications on your own. This can be dangerous. Do not hesitate to ask questions of your child's doctor. Is there any alternative? Have your child participate in the discussion and the decision if appropriate.

45. Is there any special diet or exercise that I should have my child do?

No, there is no evidence that any particular diet or exercise program has any effect on OCD. Other than following a good diet and doing regular exercise (as we all should do) there is nothing special or particular to follow in OCD.

You will see some people claim that particular diets (e.g., low carbohydrate or "natural" diets) are good for OCD. There is no evidence to support the use of any particular diet in OCD.

Similarly, you will encounter claims that exercise reduces anxiety in OCD. Although this may be true, it is not clear that this effect is anything more than the general anxiety reduction that exercise seems to bring in most individuals. That is, exercise may be a fine stress and anxiety reliever for everyone!

The Treatment—General Concepts

PART FOUR

The Treatment— Non-Drug Therapy: CBT

My son's doctor has proposed a non-drug therapy called cognitive-behavioral therapy (CBT). What is this? If OCD is a biological disorder, shouldn't it be treated with drugs?

How long does CBT take to work?

I've heard there are group treatments. I've also heard there are support groups. Are they useful, and do they work?

More . . .

46. My child's doctor has proposed a non-drug therapy called cognitive-behavioral therapy. What is this? If OCD is a biological disorder, shouldn't it be treated with drugs?

Not necessarily. Positron emission tomography (PET) scans have shown that successful behavioral treatment of OCD results in the same kinds of changes in the brain that medication can produce.

Cognitive-behavioral therapy (CBT)

A psychotherapy based on cognition (awareness), assumptions, beliefs, evaluations, and behaviors. (See Glossary for extended definition.).

Cognitive-behavioral therapy (CBT) works by helping the patient understand thoughts and beliefs that are irrational, bizarre, or inappropriate. These thoughts and perceptions lead to negative reactions, emotions, and moods that are destructive to the patient. CBT attempts to break this chain of negativity by showing how these thoughts are inaccurate, distorted, and destructive. The attempt is to then replace them with useful, realistic, and helpful thoughts and then improved behaviors.

CBT is the psychotherapy of choice for children and adolescents with OCD because it is very logical, concrete, and practical.

CBT is the psychotherapy of choice for children and adolescents with OCD because it is very logical, concrete, and practical. CBT helps the patient internalize a strategy for resisting OCD that will be of lifelong benefit. The therapist will use and adapt techniques that are appropriate for your child's developmental age.

CBT has been divided into two forms. The first is CBT that relies primarily on behavioral techniques, such as ERP (exposure and response prevention). The second is CBT that relies primarily on cognitive (thinking) techniques, such as CT (cognitive therapy), which identifies, challenges, and modifies faulty beliefs.

CBT requires motivation on the part of your child and you, the parents (who are the support system), as the techniques learned during therapy sessions must be used daily at home and integrated into your child's life and behavior.

The techniques are safe and have no real side effects. However, they may take some time (weeks to months) to start showing results.

47. I heard there is an alternative to CBT called exposure and response prevention. Is this better for my child? How is it different?

Exposure and response prevention (ERP), which actually is a type of CBT, involves gradually learning to tolerate the anxiety associated with not performing the ritual behavior.

Exposure means confronting the fear, such as touching an object felt to be contaminated. This technique is more helpful in decreasing anxieties and obsessions (e.g., fear of germs). Response prevention means not engaging in the ritual, such as not washing hands unnecessarily. This technique is more helpful in decreasing the compulsive behavior that you want to eliminate (e.g., hand washing). The therapy is based on the assumption that rituals reduce anxiety in the short-term through negative reinforcement, escaping, and/or avoiding distress.

For example, when fear of contamination causes excess hand washing, the ritual may be refusing to take a tissue from a box of tissues if the box has been touched by someone else and then washing the hands after taking the tissue. To treat this, the response prevention would be not washing the hands, knowing that this disallowance of the ritual will increase the child's level of anxiety and then helping the child to tolerate this anxiety. The child fairly quickly habituates to the anxiety-provoking situation and discovers that the level of anxiety actually drops over time. Then, by progressively increasing the level of "contamination"—that is, the length of time from taking the tissue from the box until being allowed to wash the hands—the child will see a decrease in anxiety symptoms.

Such a technique may have a place in your child's treatment plan. Be sure to discuss this option with the therapist.

> **Exposure and response prevention (ERP)**
>
> A treatment method based on the idea that a therapeutic effect is achieved as subjects confront their fears and discontinue their escape response.

48. What is the difference between the cognitive and behavioral parts of CBT? Can we do one without the other, or are they always done together?

The behavioral approach (ERP), as noted in the previous question, involves taking actions such as preventing hand washing or lengthening the time until hand washing is allowed.

Cognitive therapy (CT) is the other approach and is often added to ERP to help reduce the catastrophic thinking and exaggerated sense of responsibility often seen in children with OCD.

Cognitive therapy is non-behavioral and involves an interaction between the therapist and the patient in which the underlying thinking mechanisms, information handling, and concept formation are examined and questioned. The child is pushed to examine the way he or she handles information, develops concepts, and comes to conclusions. This type of therapy is called psychotherapy or "talk therapy" and is quite different from **behavioral therapy**. It leads to the child ultimately understanding how his or her thoughts and obsessional beliefs are not normal. Using CT can help and complement behavioral therapy (ERP). It is a therapy coming from two different directions, one behavioral (using actions) the other mental (realigning thinking and assumptions)

For example, a child may believe his healthy mother might die at work and therefore feel the need to call her there incessantly. CT will help the child to challenge the faulty assumption in this obsession. It teaches the child how to "talk back" to the obsessions, helping the child to recognize and reframe the fears in a realistic manner. Then, the child will be better able to engage in ERP (staying longer and longer periods of time with the unpleasant feelings of his mother "at risk" of dying). He will be able to avoid calling her for longer periods and ultimately will not have to call her at all.

Cognitive therapy (CT)

A type of psychotherapy in which the therapist seeks to identify and change distorted or unrealistic ways of thinking, and therefore to influence emotion and behavior.

Behavioral therapy

A type of non-drug treatment aimed at changing overt behavior by a variety of techniques, such as systematic desensitization, relaxation training, flooding, participant modeling, and positive and negative reinforcement.

49. Are there any other CBT techniques?

Yes, but they are generally less effective. These techniques include:

Thought stopping: The child is taught to recognize the start of the fear and to make an effort to stop the negative thoughts.

Distraction: As soon as the obsessive thought starts, the child starts doing a pleasant activity.

Satiation: This technique involves listening to a prolonged discussion about the obsession, often presented by an audio recording. For example, the child may listen to a tape that discusses germs. The theory here is that the mind becomes so saturated with the subject that the fear decreases.

Habit reversal: This technique involves replacing an OCD ritual by another behavior that does not belong to the ritual. Again, to use the fear of germs as an example, the child would be instructed to take a pen and write something rather than washing his or her hands.

Contingency management: This technique uses rewards and punishment to prevent the ritual. Using the germ example, a point system can be put in place. For each time the ritual is blocked by not washing the hands, the child is rewarded with a point. When a certain number of points that week is reached, the child receives a special treat such as ice cream or going to a movie.

50. What are the advantages of CBT? Is it painful or difficult?

CBT is basically free of side effects other than some anxiety during the treatment. The therapist will grade the child's symptoms and start slowly with the easiest one. The therapist will develop a hierarchy of situations that the child avoids (this is called a "fear-ladder") and will design small challenges that will teach the child to delay compulsions for short periods of time and then for increasingly longer periods. The child is in control of the treatment even if it is hard work. It is a treatment that is logical and as experience has shown, very effective. When successful, the rewards are enormous. Children who respond to this treatment often stay well for long periods of time.

CBT can be used alone or combined with medications. It can prevent relapses when medications are stopped and can increase the response to the medications if they are only partially effective. Children (or parents) who refuse medication can use this treatment. It can be used any time: before the medication treatment, during, or after. Therapy must be adapted to the child's developmental level.

In severe cases, the psychiatrist may recommend hospitalization of the child because several treatments a day may be needed at the beginning. In most cases, however, outpatient treatment is very effective and quite sufficient. Visits may be more frequent at the beginning (e.g., 2 or 3 times a week), decreasing over time. In successful cases, three maintenance visits per year may be sufficient.

51. My son was told he should not have CBT as the first treatment. Why not? Why drugs right away? Can we use CBT later, and are there times when CBT isn't the best treatment?

Ideally, CBT can and should be started right away. However, some children are too severely impaired by the symptoms of OCD and may require medications first to lessen the symptoms in order to benefit from CBT later on.

CBT is time consuming and has to be done regularly. Some children or parents do not want to face the work and anxiety associated with the treatment.

About 25% of children and/or parents refuse CBT. The child and parents have to be motivated participants, and some are not able to commit to this therapy. CBT is time consuming and has to be done regularly. Some children or parents do not want to face the work and anxiety associated with the treatment. And finally, it is sometimes impossible to find a therapist trained in CBT in that area.

52. How do I find a behavioral therapist?

Here are some methods for locating a behavioral therapist:

- Ask your psychiatrist or someone in the local mental health clinic.
- Contact the psychiatry, psychology, or social work department at a local university medical center.
- Contact the local OCD support group.
- Contact the Obsessive Compulsive Foundation (http://www.ocfoundation.org), the Anxiety Disorders Association of America (http://www.adaa.org), or the Association for Behavioral and Cognitive Therapies (http://www.aabt.org).

And of course, recommendations from satisfied parents of children with OCD in support groups may be very helpful. You should avoid making your choice based only on advertisements in the phone book or local advertising flyers.

A behavioral therapist does not have to be a physician. In fact, most of them are not. They can be psychiatrists, psychologists, social workers, and licensed mental health workers, such as nurses or counselors who have received the specialized training.

Although the treatment is very popular, effective, and widely used, you may still need to travel to a treatment center that specializes in intensive CBT. In addition, not all insurance companies will reimburse well or fully for CBT.

Finally, it is possible that a psychiatrist or a therapist you would like to work with might be willing to learn the skills involved in CBT. Most therapists have had some level of basic CBT therapy during their training.

53. How long does CBT take to work? Will I see improvement as we go along? Where should CBT be done? What else should I know about CBT?

When sessions are given weekly, CBT may take 2 months or more to become effective. In intensive CBT, usually given in 2- to 3-hour daily sessions, it may become effective in as little as 3 weeks of treatment. The intensity of the treatment and its effectiveness depend on the severity of the symptoms, the motivation of the child and parents, and whether the techniques are used by the child and family at home.

Most often, therapy is done in the therapist's office with daily homework (that is, using the techniques taught by the therapist). Homework is critical because the exercises are carried out at the time and place that trigger the obsessions and compulsions. The exercises are tailored to the child's problems and severity.

In some intensive CBT, the therapist may initially come to the child's home to do the practice. In very severe cases, the child may require initial treatment in a hospital setting.

It is important to note that studies in adults and children with OCD show that CBT is not effective in all patients, and its efficacy can depend on the approach used. ERP (exposure and response prevention) conducted by a therapist is better than ERP guided by a computer and a guide book. Those who complete the treatment report a 50% to 80% reduction in OCD symptoms after 12 to 20 sessions. Patients who respond to treatment usually stay well for several years. This therapy seems superior to medication alone.

Several factors affect the outcome of ERP. These factors include the child's adherence to the treatment, the degree of insight into the irrationality of the fears, and presence of other conditions at the same time, such as depression or other anxiety disorders. Incorporating relapse-prevention procedures into ERP appears to improve the long-term outcome.

CBT alone, whether done individually or in a group, has helped children to maintain their progress at a 6-month follow-up. CBT can be used alone in many cases and has been shown effective in producing symptom improvement and sometimes complete remission. It is also very useful in treating relapses. When the techniques are adopted by the child and the family, they can be carried out at home without waiting for an appointment with the therapist.

54. Our daughter finally has gotten better. Her symptoms are minimal now or nearly all gone. How can we prevent relapses?

Congratulations! This success no doubt required much work on your daughter's and your part. Now you should concentrate on relapse prevention procedures.

First, you, your daughter, and the therapist should assess the stressors likely to trigger the OCD symptoms. The techniques and strategies used to resist compulsions and obsessions should be continued either in the same manner or in a manner proposed by your therapist. The family must remain observant and supportive.

Obviously, continuation of the successful initial treatments, good nutrition, sleep, and exercise will lessen the likelihood of reverses. The homework taught by the therapist should be continued, as should the regular visits to the therapist (even if only 2 or 3 times a year). Medication, if prescribed, should not be stopped unless the physician agrees.

Other techniques, which may or may not have been used during the acute treatment, may be used. These techniques include:

> *Cognitive treatment*: This treatment involves targeting dysfunctional beliefs (such as the overestimation of danger and an inflated personal sense of responsibility) and using techniques to combat them. This treatment

is very similar to the techniques used during the initial, acute phase of CBT.

Associative therapy: This technique may involve free association about OCD symptoms combined with progressive muscle relaxation (PMR) therapy. Speak to your therapist about this approach.

Everybody involved should realize that prevention of relapses is a long-term affair and that there will likely be occasional setbacks and relapses.

Everybody involved (patient, parents, family, friends, school, and other support) should realize that prevention of relapses is a long-term affair and that there will likely be occasional setbacks and relapses. The goal is to catch them early and minimize their severity when they do occur. As with most everything in medicine, it is easier and better to prevent something from occurring than to treat it after it has happened. As you can see, parents and siblings can have a major impact on the child's treatment by encouraging progress, helping with the homework, not participating in the rituals, providing suggestions for rewards, and providing reassurance.

55. I've heard there are group treatments. I've also heard there are support groups. Are they useful, and do they work?

Yes, these groups do exist. Only limited studies have been done to answer whether they are useful and effective. The data seems to show that the response to treatment is faster with individual behavioral therapy than with group therapy.

Group therapy ERP is useful for less severe OCD. From the public health point of view, group therapy is more "efficient," as one therapist can treat multiple patients at the same time, leaving more time to help the more severe cases individually. It may also be less expensive for the patient and family than individual therapy.

Support groups are very useful, as they provide understanding and mutual acceptance. People can develop a sense of camaraderie with other attendees who have struggled through the same difficulties. Helpful strategies are frequently discussed.

Bottom line: Support groups and multifamily sessions are useful but probably not sufficient if used in place of standard treatments by a skilled practitioner.

56. What is multifamily CBT? I heard I would be a "co-therapist" for my daughter. I'm not trained at all in this, and I'm not sure I could do it. Could you explain?

Multifamily CBT is treatment given in a group format. Patients accompanied by one or two family members attend usually weekly sessions to learn about the disorder (psychoeducation) and the behavioral techniques used to treat the symptoms. They learn how to practice these techniques at home. The education provided by the therapist is adapted to the content and the needs of the group. Time is given to members to practice so they will be able to reproduce this at home. Time is also given for members to share their experiences and ask questions. With some time, a parent may be able to co-lead the group with the therapist and help other children and parents going through some of the difficult times they went through themselves.

Multifamily CBT has shown to be effective. In one study where a family member functioned as a co-therapist in the treatment group, patients improved significantly more than when no family member was a co-therapist.

PART FIVE

The Treatment— Medications

What are the drugs used to treat OCD?

How quickly will the SSRI work in my son?
How long should treatment be given?

How will the doctor choose which medication to give my child?

My child has not responded well to any of the medications that usually work in OCD. Are there any other medications that can be tried?

More . . .

57. What drugs are used to treat OCD?

Serotonin reuptake inhibitors (SRIs)

Drugs that increase the level of serotonin in the synapses but are not selective and have some actions on other neurotransmitters as well. They are used in the treatment of OCD and other disorders like depression.

Serotonin reuptake inhibitors (SRIs) are the only clearly effective medications for OCD in children. Although many drugs have been tried over the years, this is the only class of drugs with strong scientific evidence of effectiveness. They work by increasing the concentration of serotonin, a chemical messenger implicated in the cause of OCD, in the brain.

The medications prevent serotonin from being taken back into the original neuron that released it (see Questions 8 and 58). Instead, serotonin can then bind to the receptor sites of the nearby target neurons and send chemical messages or signals that can help regulate the excessive anxiety and the obsessive thoughts. Thus, the drugs are believed to function by increasing the serotonin taken up by the receptor nerve cell, which decreases the anxiety and obsessions.

Five drugs are approved by the FDA for treatment of OCD in the United States. These five are all serotonin uptake inhibitors (SRIs). Four of them are selective serotonin uptake inhibitors (SSRIs): fluoxetine (Prozac), fluvoxamine (Luvox), paroxetine (Paxil), and sertraline (Zoloft). As with all drugs, each has two names; the first listed is the generic name, and the second (in parentheses) is the brand name. These medications are called "selective" because they act primarily on serotonin and not on other neurotransmitters. By being selective, they are felt to be more specific to serotonin-related diseases and have fewer side effects.

Antidepressants

Medicines used to stop depression; they are non-addictive (e.g., SSRIs like Prozac, TCAs like Anafranil).

Non-selective serotonin inhibitors act on multiple neurotransmitters (such as serotonin and norepinephrine) at the same time. Although this less-regulated effect means they may have wider ranges of use, they may also be less specific and produce more unwanted side effects. One of these drugs, clomipramine (Anafranil), is approved for OCD in the United States. This drug is older and appears to have more side effects. Although FDA-approved for OCD, it is not a first choice for treatment. These drugs are also used to treat depression and are called "**antidepressants.**"

58. How well do these selective and non-selective serotonin drugs work? What are the side effects?

The four SSRIs approved in the United States for treating OCD all appear to be equally effective.

Fluvoxamine (Luvox) is proven effective in treating OCD. The most frequent side effects are insomnia, nausea, and somnolence. There are fewer anticholinergic effects (e.g., dry mouth, constipation, urinary problems) and sexual dysfunctions than with clomipramine. A slow release form of Luvox (Luvox XR) to be given once a day just came out on the market but has not been approved by the FDA for treating OCD in children. The FDA-approved **labeling** for Luvox describes a study in children in which improvement occurred in 76% of those treated with Luvox compared to a 50% improvement in children given **placebo**. Of the children showing improvement with Luvox, 39% were very much or much improved.

Fluoxetine (Prozac) has also shown good efficacy and good tolerability even at high doses.

Sertraline (Zoloft) is comparable in efficacy and tolerability to the other SSRIs mentioned here. Side effects can occur, including nervousness, upset stomach, or insomnia.

A recent large-scale multisite, randomized, placebo-controlled trial of CBT, sertraline (Zoloft), and a combination of CBT and sertraline in children with OCD was performed (called The Pediatric OCD Treatment Study [POTS]). The results showed that both CBT alone and sertraline alone were superior to placebo (sugar pills). Better symptom reduction was found in patients receiving CBT in combination with sertraline.

The Treatment—Medications

Labeling

When referring to a drug, the FDA-approved documentation describing the use, dose, side effects, warnings, etc., for a drug.

Placebo reaction

When a person has a positive effect from an innocuous substance such as a sugar pill.

Paroxetine (Paxil) is used in treating OCD, but rarely in children. It is an effective medication. The evidence suggests that it is more likely to induce more side effects such as weight gain than the other SSRIs. Also, it carries a greater risk of an unpleasant **withdrawal** syndrome, so when used it must be stopped very slowly

Withdrawal

The psychological and or physical reaction to abruptly stopping a dependence-producing drug.

The clinical studies on these drugs in children are relatively few compared to adults. The results in general suggest that higher doses work better than lower doses (though higher doses may produce more side effects). The results are similar with all the drugs, with symptoms very much improved in 7% to 20% of patients, much improved in 18% to 24%, and minimally improved in 29% to 39%. Placebo responses were lower and ranged from around 7% to 24%. Thus, based on the studies cited in the FDA's labeling, the majority of children had some level of improvement.

Children with oppositional defiant disorder have been shown to have the lowest improvement rate in trials with paroxetine and were not likely to be as successful in CBT trials unless pretreatment with parent training had occurred.

Augmentation strategies

Used in clinical practice when patients fail to achieve remission on one medicine. At that point, another medicine may be added to increase the action of the first one.

The non-selective drug clomipramine (Anafranil) was first approved by the FDA in 1989 and is used for the treatment of OCD in the United States. It is an effective treatment. However, adverse effects have been reported, especially dry mouth (a problem if the child has orthodontic braces), constipation, weight gain, low blood pressure, irregular heartbeat, somnolence, and sexual dysfunctions (in adolescents). There may also be effects on liver enzymes, and there is a potential for seizures at high doses. Laboratory tests may be necessary as well as an electrocardiogram before and during treatment. Due to these problems, it is not the first line of treatment but can be used if the other medications do not work. Clomipramine may also be used as an **augmentation** agent with other treatments. Due to the danger of seizures and heart problems, many physicians obtain a blood level to ensure that it falls within a safe range.

Table 6   Approved Drugs for OCD

Drug	Age Use	Typical Starting Dosage (mg/day)	Daily Dose (mg/day)	Formulations Available
Fluvoxamine (Luvox)	Children >8 years old	12.5–25	12.5-200	Tabs 25, 50, 100, 150 mg Extended-release exists (only approved in adults) Generic exists
Fluoxetine (Prozac)	Children >6 years old	5	25-60	Tabs 10 mg Capsules 10, 20, 40 mg Oral solution 20 mg/5 mL Generic exists
Sertraline (Zoloft)	Children >7 years old	12.5–25	25-200	Tabs 25, 50, 100 mg Oral solution 20 mg/mL Generic exists
Paroxetine (Paxil)	Patients >18 years old	10	20-60	Tabs 10, 20, 30, 40 mg Oral suspension 10 mg/5 mL Controlled release formulation also exists Generic exists
Chlomipramine (Anafranil)	Children >10 years old	12.5–25	25-200	Caps 25, 50, 75 mg Generic exists

Although these medications are effective in many patients, only about one patient in five will be free of OCD symptoms with drug treatment alone. Most patients will need combination treatment with medication and CBT to achieve more complete and lasting results.

Most patients will need combination treatment with medication and CBT to achieve more complete and lasting results.

59. Wait a minute, these are antidepressant drugs. My son isn't depressed. He has OCD. Why are antidepressants being used for OCD?

These five medications are also approved for the treatment of depression and anxiety disorders and are commonly referred to as "antidepressants." These drugs are used for depression and other disorders because they are felt to be serotonin-based disorders also. Obviously, depression and anxiety disorders are quite different from OCD. There are many areas of all these diseases that are not well understood. But based on research in the lab and in patients, it is clear that drugs that act on the serotonin systems are effective in a variety of disorders.

60. What doses are used? Are they dangerous? Are they higher than doses for other problems?

The doses used in OCD are higher than the doses used in depression and generalized anxiety. Frequently, the higher the dose, the higher the possibility of side effects. These drugs are better tolerated when started at low doses and then increased progressively as needed to reach the best level of effectiveness.

These drugs should be decreased gradually before being totally stopped to prevent withdrawal symptoms—particularly if high doses are being used. Obviously, these drugs must be used with great care, and any changes in the doses or in the timing should be discussed with the treating physician.

Often, not much improvement is seen with the first SSRI used, and a different one will need to be tried. Overall, the medications are effective in about 40% to 60% of patients. As noted in Question 58, only about one patient in five will become free of OCD symptoms with drug treatment alone, but the data does suggest that improvement will be seen in more than 50% of the patients with drug treatment.

Anti-OCD medications control symptoms but do not cure the disorder. Therefore, the positive effects of the medication occur only as long as the medicine is being taken. If some symptoms remain, their intensity may be lessened. At this point, there is no known cure for OCD.

If none of the approved medications work, the psychiatrist may want to try higher doses of the approved drugs, combinations of drugs, or using drugs that are approved by the FDA for other diseases but not for OCD. These medication decisions, of course, should be done with great caution and with continued close surveillance of the child.

61. How quickly will the SSRI work in my son? How long should treatment be given?

Unfortunately, all anti-OCD medications work slowly. They are not a "quick fix" but should be considered as part of the long-term treatment program.

When patients are asked how well they are doing on medication compared to before treatment, they usually report moderate to marked improvement after about 8 to 12 weeks of treatment. If an improvement is seen after several weeks, it is recommended that the dose be maintained for at least about 10 weeks before dose escalation is considered. However, once the highest dose is reached, it is best to continue for at least 3 months at this level. Improvement may continue over the next several months (or even up to a year) with long-term continuation of the medication at the same dose.

It is important for you and your son to understand up front about the delay before a response is seen. You should understand that your son may need a long period on the medication before it appears to work. You should resist the urge to rapidly increase the dose prematurely.

Unfortunately, side effects often do not take a long time to occur; you may see them very quickly after a dose is increased. These side effects are another reason not to risk a rapid increase in dose. Should side effects occur after a dose increase, your child's physician may have to stop the drug (which would not have occurred if the lower dose had been maintained). Alternatively, if the side effect is not severe, the physician may elect to decrease the dose rather than stopping the drug. The rule is to taper very slowly over many months while adding behavioral therapy to prevent relapse.

Depending on how well symptoms respond and what other treatments are used, the physician may propose drug treatment to be given for 1 to 2 years, or sometimes longer. Each child's treatment is individualized in terms of dose and duration. The response cannot be predicted in advance. Many patients want to stay on medication due to its benefits.

62. What other drugs are used, even if unapproved by the FDA?

Other drugs have been used but mostly with adults. Their application in children is very limited.

Other antidepressants such as citalopram (Celexa), escitalopram (Lexapro), mirtazapine (Remeron), and venlafaxine (Effexor) have been tried with some good results. **Tricyclic antidepressants** other than clomipramine have been tried but have shown no evidence of efficacy in the treatment of OCD. Why this is the case is not understood.

Tricyclic antidepressants (TCAs)

Among the first types of medication used to treat depression; popular before SSRIs came into wide use; can be used to treat panic disorder.

Monoamine oxidase inhibitors (MAOIs) are an old class of drugs used to treat depression. They have largely been replaced by the newer antidepressants (SSRIs). MAOIs can produce severe side effects such as cardiovascular problems and weight gain. They also have major interactions with other drugs, and some medications (such as fluoxetine) need to be stopped at least 5 weeks before starting MAOIs. These interactions along with the severe dietary restrictions required when using them have made their use extremely rare, particularly with children.

Monoamine oxidase inhibitors (MAOIs)

A standard medication for panic attacks. They work by stopping the breakdown of monoamines (like serotonin and norepinephrine) by irreversibly inhibiting the enzyme monoamine oxidase.

Other therapies used without medically proven efficacy, and with significant risk in many cases, include **benzodiazepines**, high-dose minerals and vitamins, St. John's wort, antipsychotic drugs, narcotics, and experimental drugs. You may see lots of claims on the Internet for these and other unproven products. Be very careful. You should discuss with your child's doctor any additional treatment you might want to begin.

Benzodiazepines

A type of drug used for short-term treatment of panic attacks to decrease anxiety; potentially addictive.

63. How will the doctor choose which medication to give my child?

The SSRIs are the first-line drugs to treat OCD because of their established efficacy and safety. The benefits of treatment clearly outweigh the risks. The issue is how to select among them, as all appear equally efficacious in treating OCD. The choice is based upon the *side effect profile* of a particular SSRI and the presence of particular *comorbid conditions* in the given patient. The choice may also depend upon **drug interactions**.

For example, paroxetine (Paxil) and fluoxetine (Prozac) raise the blood levels of most antipsychotics and beta-blockers that some patients might also be taking. Fluvoxamine (Luvox) also increases the level of some antipsychotic medications such as olanzapine (Zyprexa).

Some other considerations include:

- Effectiveness of a particular drug in another family member or in the child, if used in the past
- The psychiatrist's prior successes or experience with a particular drug
- Concerns about the child's risk of overdosing (there is more risk of lethality with tricyclic antidepressants)
- The cost of the medication or its availability, if managed care or insurance is involved
- The FDA approval status of the drug, if an unapproved drug is proposed

As with many related drugs in the same chemical class, some children (or adults) who do not respond to one SSRI may respond to another. There is no way to predict who responds to which drug and no data to help decide what the next drug should be. If two or three trials of SSRIs fail, then it may be worth considering the non-selective clomipramine (Anafranil) next.

If all the SSRIs and clomipramine fail to work well, the physician should then consider other non-FDA-approved drugs, realizing that data is not available and that there may be greater risks than with the approved and better-studied drugs. The treating physician should have experience with the use

Drug (or drug–drug) interaction

When two or more drugs are given together and interfere with each other, possibly producing side effects or decreasing the effectiveness of one or more of the drugs.

The Treatment—Medications

of unapproved drugs in OCD in children. He or she may ask you to sign an informed consent indicating that the risks and issues have been explained to you and your child.

64. When should we consider medication for our daughter with OCD?

Medication should be considered when children are experiencing significant distress or impairment that disturbs normal life. It should also be considered when CBT is unavailable or only partially effective.

Very mild cases generally will not need medication. Mild cases may need only CBT. However, if the symptoms become more severe, you and your daughter should seek professional help to confirm the diagnosis and discuss treatment options. More severe cases may require medications and CBT. Each child is different, and there are no clear generalities beyond these that apply.

Metabolism

The body's reaction to a medication; faster in some than in others. Thus, people can require different doses of the same medication to receive similar effects.

As many pharmacologists and physicians state: Children are not just small adults. They may respond differently to medications than do adults.

If, on the other hand, your daughter is already under professional care for her OCD and the symptoms seem to be severe or worsening, or if the trial of non-drug therapy has been sufficiently long to say that it has not helped adequately (that is, the symptoms are still troublesome and disturbing normal life), then you should discuss medication therapy with your daughter's physician—if he or she has not brought the subject up already.

65. Will my child's response to the medication be different from an adult's response?

Yes, that is very possible. As many pharmacologists and physicians state: Children are not just small adults. They may respond differently to medications than do adults.

Children often **metabolize** and eliminate drugs more quickly than adults. This rapid processing means that children may have to be given higher doses and may necessitate the use of "adult-size" doses in order to produce good therapeutic effects.

In addition, each person may respond differently to the same dose of a drug, so treatment plans and doses must be tailored to the individual patient. The dose used of any drug should be the smallest dose that effectively treats your child's OCD. Once your child is getting effective treatment, it is not necessarily true that "if some is good, more is better."

There can be different effects in children of different ages with the same dose of a drug because the central nervous system is at different stages of development compared to adults, where development has reached maturity. That is, a 40-year-old and a 45-year-old will probably react in a similar manner to the same drug, but a 2-year-old will probably not react the same way as a 7-year-old. No two children respond to anti-OCD medication in the same way. Sometimes a child will not respond to any medication, and sometimes a child will respond differently to each of the anti-OCD medications. The only way to know is to try the drug in the child.

The occurrence of side effects varies a lot from one medication to another, as well as from one child to another. For example, adolescents have a higher risk of **dystonic** side effects to certain antipsychotic drugs (i.e., narcoleptics) than do adults. Prepubertal children are at a higher risk for the activating side-effects (e.g., agitation, insomnia) of SSRIs. Undesirable behavioral side effects (separate from the improvement in the OCD behaviors) have been described. They can occur with any of the anti-OCD drugs and are characterized by a significant change in the child's behavior. Parents have said that their child became "too happy or silly" or "oppositional and defiant." Increased aggressiveness has also been seen.

Dystonia
A brain disease in which muscles contract and produce repetitive, irregular spasms and twisting or abnormal postures.

Most of the time, these changes are mild and go away without the need to modify the treatment. If the side effects are a problem and need to be addressed, reducing the dose of the medication is often sufficient, particularly if the lower dose worked in the past without the side effect. Alternatively, stopping this drug and switching to an alternative medication may work.

The Treatment—Medications

66. My son can't take pills very well. Are there liquid forms of these drugs?

Some children have difficulty swallowing pills (tablets or capsules). Some of the medicines exist in liquid form. An alternative would be to crush a tablet between two spoons or to pull apart and empty a gelatin capsule. The medicine can then be added to some apple sauce or jelly. Before doing this, however, check with your pharmacist, since some drugs are made in long-acting formulations that must not be crushed or cut.

Lower dosages should be used in young children and children with neuro-developmental disorders.

67. What about generic drugs. Are they okay? How about drugs from Internet pharmacies?

Generic medication

A drug that contains the same active ingredient(s) as the name brand, though the inactive ingredients (e.g., fillers), shape, color, preservatives, and packaging may be different.

Broadly speaking, the FDA has indicated that the **generic drugs** it has approved are "safe and effective." Because many of them come from outside the United States, some questions have arisen about their quality. Discuss these drugs with your physician or pharmacist.

Internet drugs, however, are a different story if you cannot be sure where they are from. It is very unwise to purchase OCD medications online and to give these drugs to your child. A physician should always examine your child and prescribe the drug.

The FDA has stated:

> Patients who buy prescription drugs from Websites operating outside the law are at increased risk of suffering life-threatening adverse events, such as side effects from inappropriately prescribed medications, dangerous drug interactions, contaminated drugs, and impure or unknown ingredients found in unapproved drugs . . . The Internet makes it easy for unscrupulous

people to sell drugs to patients without these safeguards in place. A Website may appear to be associated with a legitimate pharmacy when in fact it is not. Websites that sell prescription drugs without a valid prescription deny consumers the protection provided by an examination conducted by a licensed practitioner.

If you wish to read the FDA's complete review of this subject, visit the FDA Web site at http://www.fda.gov/oc/buyonline/faqs.html.

68. What should I do if my son's physician wants to use a drug that is not FDA approved to treat his OCD? Should I allow this?

In general, before considering the use of a non-approved drug, the ones that are approved should be tried first. Some children will not be helped by one or two of the drugs but will be helped by one of the others.

There are other SSRIs approved by the FDA for depression or other diseases but not OCD. Although it is possible that they would work in your child, the lack of approval suggests there is insufficient data or experience with this drug in treating OCD. It may also mean that tests were never done in children with this drug so no information is available even in the medical literature.

Keep in mind also that clomipramine, the non-selective serotonin inhibitor, has been added to an SSRI with a positive effect in some children. This combination should be considered by your son's physician also.

If, after all of these efforts, your son's physician does want to try an unapproved drug, this option should be considered. You should discuss the option with your son's physician and be sure you and the physician understand the possible benefits and risks of the drug, particularly if it is of a different class from the SSRIs. Your son's physician may have extensive experience using unapproved drugs with good results (especially if he or she is at a major research medical center), and this past experience should be taken into account. Obviously, your son should be very closely monitored when using any new drug.

69. I've heard these drugs can increase the risk of suicide. What must I watch for?

These drugs have a "black box" warning about the possibility of worsening suicidal thoughts.

The FDA warning for the drugs is shown in Figure 6.

Thus, thoughts and behaviors suggestive of self-harm or suicide must be carefully monitored, particularly at the initiation of the medications and when doses are increased.

Thus, thoughts and behaviors suggestive of self-harm or suicide must be carefully monitored, particularly at the initiation of the medications and when doses are increased.

Antidepressants increased the risk of suicidal thinking and behavior (suicidality) in short-term studies in children and adolescents with Major Depressive Disorder (MDD) and other psychiatric disorders. Anyone considering the use of [Insert established name] or any other antidepressant in a child or adolescent must balance this risk with the clinical need. Patients who are started on therapy should be observed closely for clinical worsening, suicidality, or unusual changes in behavior. Families and caregivers should be advised of the need for close observation and communication with the prescriber. [Insert established name] is not approved for use in pediatric patients. (See Warnings and Precautions: Pediatric Use) [This sentence would be revised to reflect if a drug were approved for a pediatric indication(s). Such as, [Insert established name] is not approved for use in pediatric patients except for patients with [Insert approved pediatric indication(s)]. (See Warnings and Precautions: Pediatric Use)]

Figure 6   FDA Warning of Suicidality in Children and Adolescents

70. My child is taking an SSRI. What side effects should I look for in my child, and how do I handle them?

The most common side effects include gastrointestinal distress (including pain, nausea, vomiting, and diarrhea). Headaches, tremor, agitation, and nervousness may also be seen. These side effects can be minimized by starting with lower doses. Usually, they disappear by themselves. Of course, not every patient has side effects, and not every patient who does have side effects has all of them.

Other side effects that may occur include:

Insomnia: If insomnia occurs, it may be more useful to have your child take the medication in the morning rather than the evening. In extreme cases, a sleeping pill could be used, but it should not be used chronically.

Sweating: Sweating can be treated with low doses of anticholinergic agents such as benztropine mesylate (Cogentin).

Sexual side effects: These may affect up to one-third of adolescents taking SSRIs. Adolescents will not talk spontaneously about this, so the physician should ask specifically. Management includes reducing the SSRI dose.

In many cases, the side effect will disappear on its own with no treatment and without having to stop the medication. Sometimes it is useful to switch to a different SSRI that may have the same effectiveness but not the side effects.

Another rare but serious side effect seen with the use of SSRIs and if other serotoninergic drugs are used at the same time is the serotonin syndrome. This side effect is usually seen within 24 hours of starting the medication or changing the dose. It can also be seen with overdoses. Symptoms include nausea, diarrhea, chills, sweating, dizziness, elevated temperature, elevated blood pressure, tremor, agitation, exaggerated reflexes, muscle twitches, and confusion. Serotonin syndrome is a medical emergency, and you should stop all medicines, contact your child's physician, and get the child to an emergency room immediately. It may progress to seizures, coma, and death if untreated.

71. If my son is on an SSRI and we and the doctor decide to stop the medication, is there anything to watch out for? Can it just be stopped all at once, or should we gradually lower the dose?

The drug should be gradually stopped. If not, your child is at risk for a drug discontinuation syndrome. This syndrome may be seen after the rapid stopping of SSRIs, particularly after paroxetine (Paxil), or serotonin-norepinephrine reuptake inhibitors (SNRIs) like venlafaxine (Effexor) or duloxetine (Cymbalta). The syndrome consists of dizziness, nausea and vomiting, headache, lethargy, agitation, insomnia, abnormal movements, and paresthesias (tingling or funny feelings).

The drug needs to be tapered down very slowly. If OCD symptoms occur with the decrease of medication, raising the medication dose and slowing down further dose reductions will be necessary.

SSRIs and SNRIs are not addictive. The discontinuation syndrome is not the same thing as the syndrome seen when an addicting drug (like an opiate) is stopped.

72. These drugs are approved for kids over 7 years of age. My daughter is 5 and has been diagnosed with OCD. Can she take one of these drugs?

Children younger than 6 years old may have OCD, although the diagnosis is difficult to make. In some cases, medications may be recommended, particularly if the child is experiencing significant disability and distress. There is little information in the medical literature regarding the use of anti-OCD medications in preschoolers. You should discuss this concern with your child's psychiatrist, and you may want to consider a second medical opinion in a difficult case such as this.

73. I've heard that if someone is taking more than one drug there can be interactions between the drugs. Is this true? What do I need to be concerned about?

Drug interactions refer to the situation when someone is taking two or more drugs at the same time. It is possible that the drugs will interfere with each other, decreasing the efficacy of one or more of them or producing increased side effects. The possibility for such interactions will always be evaluated by the physician (and the pharmacist) if the patient is taking more than one drug. It is important to be aware that combining medications of any kind, including over-the-counter ones, can produce interactions and side effects that can complicate the treatment of OCD.

It is possible that the drugs will interfere with each other, decreasing the efficacy of one or more of them or producing increased side effects.

All the medications that the child is taking should be reported to the psychiatrist and the pediatrician—including psychiatric medications, but also asthma medicines, antibiotics, over-the-counter cough medicines, anti-acne medications, and all others.

Here are two examples of drug interactions:

- Taken with fluvoxamine (Luvox), caffeine may produce sweating, nervousness, trembling, and insomnia.
- Taken with OCD medicines, dextromethorphan (e.g., Robitussin) may lead to extreme anxiety and chest and abdominal discomfort.

Some SSRIs are noted to have possible interactions with pimozide, warfarin, theophylline, certain benzodiazepines, omeprazole, and phenytoin. The use of medication combinations must be done on a case-by-case basis and after consideration of risks and benefits.

74. Does the doctor tailor the treatment to my child's special needs, or does one treatment work for everyone?

Each child with OCD must have a specific therapy program tailored for him or her. There is no "one size fits all." The choice will be made by your child's physician based on the severity of the symptoms, the duration of the disease, the age of your child, the developmental needs, the family context and support available, the availability of CBT, the effectiveness of the CBT if already tried, tolerance and allergies to medications, dosage form available (e.g., liquids, tablets), and other factors. This decision is obviously very complex, and it needs to be made by the physician with consultation with the family and other team members.

The complexity of this decision is why it is so important to seek the help of therapists who are trained to work with children and their families. It is also the reason why a child therapist will ask so many questions about family members, the home situation, the babysitting or child care situation, extended family members that the child is in contact with, whom the child is close to, whom he or she has conflicts with, the school situation, who his or her friends are, and other questions specific to your child.

With this information, the therapist will be able to put in place treatment that is individualized for your child. Younger children, having less emotional awareness and expressive skills, may require more guidance and direction from their parents. Adolescents who may struggle with some autonomy issues may look more oppositional and will need a different approach. Your child's doctor will help you determine that.

75. If my child is to take medications, are there questions to ask the doctor?

Questions you will want to ask the doctor regarding your child's medications include:

- What are the brand and generic names?
- How is this medication helpful? What is its success rate?
- How long before it starts working?
- What are the side effects?
- Is it addictive?
- What is the daily dosage? How often should it be taken during the day?
- If my child misses a dose, what do I do? Use the regular dose? Double the next dose?
- What tests need to be done before starting the medicine? And then while my child is still taking it?
- How will you monitor the response? Will you make changes in the dosage if needed?
- Which medications and what food should not be given with this medicine?
- Can my child take over-the-counter medicine with this medication?
- Any activities to be restricted because of this medicine? For example, during outdoor sports, should there be protection from the sun?
- How long will my child be on this medicine?
- What is next if this medicine is not well tolerated or does not work?
- What can I give my child if he has a headache or a virus or stomach pain?

The Treatment—Medications

- Is there a generic version available? Do the generics work as well as the branded versions, and are they as safe?
- (For the pharmacist) What is the cost difference between the generic and the brand?
- Where can I get a written list of the possible side effects?
- What are the long-term risks if my child needs to stay on this medicine for a very long time?
- Are there any very serious or life-threatening risks?
- What has happened in overdoses?
- What do I watch for about the suicide risk?
- Ask any additional questions you have about your child's medication.

In summary: Be sure to take the time to ask these questions and be sure you understand the answers. Your doctor should be able to provide information that not only makes you feel more comfortable with your child's medication but also enables you to administer it appropriately.

76. My child has not responded well to any of the medications that usually work in OCD. Are there any other medications that can be tried?

Yes, but most of the experience is in adults. Unfortunately, there is not a lot of research done in children for most drugs—both psychiatric drugs and other drugs—for lots of reasons. The FDA and the drug companies are working to increase research, and it is now being done more and more in children, but it still lags behind what is tested in adults.

Here are some of the other drugs sometimes tried in OCD. Again, it must be emphasized that these are not approved by the FDA for use in OCD, and some of them are not even approved at all in the United States (e.g., hallucinogens). Some are not regulated by the FDA as they are considered food supplements or nutritionals and not drugs.

- Other SRIs, including sertraline (Zoloft), citalopram (Celexa), and escitalopram (Lexapro) have been used in OCD but are not FDA approved.
- Pindolol, a beta-blocker (normally used for high blood pressure) has been used a few times with some success as an augmentation agent. The greatest improvement was noted in the ability to resist compulsions.
- Benzodiazepines such as diazepam (Valium), lorazepam (Ativan), alprazolam (Xanax), and others have been used at modest doses to relieve anxiety and distress but do not change obsessions and compulsions. They cannot be recommended as monotherapy for OCD, as they can be addictive if used for long periods of time.
- Buspirone (Buspar), a non-benzodiazepine anti-anxiety drug, has shown inconsistent results when used in OCD. It has been tried in children and adolescents as combined therapy with an SSRI (useful in adolescents as a combined treatment with SSRIs at a dose of 20 mg/day).
- Inositol is found in the body as well as in many foods and has been tried in OCD. It has been recommended by alternative medicine Web sites. There is no clear evidence of its usefulness.
- Lithium is a drug used for the treatment of **bipolar** (manic depressive) **disorders**. It is not effective in treating OCD but is used if there is also a bipolar disorder in a child with OCD.
- Narcotics such as morphine sulfate and narcotic-like drugs such as tramadol have been tried for resistant OCD. Problems include sedation and **addiction** in long-term use.
- Anticonvulsant medications such as topiramate and lamotrigine have been reported to be useful in some cases either as monotherapy or as augmentation agents.
- D-amphetamine has been reported to have an acute anti-OCD effect in some cases.

Bipolar disorder

A mood disorder where the person experiences both an elated state (hypomania or mania) and at other times depression.

Addiction

A pattern of drug abuse characterized by compulsive use of the drug, excessive focus on getting a supply of the drug, and a high likelihood of relapse when the drug use is stopped.

- Hallucinogens such as psilocybin have been reported to alleviate OCD in individual cases but are not recommended. They are not considered therapeutic drugs, and most are illegal or very tightly controlled.
- St. John's wort has been tried without success and was associated with side effects such as photosensitivity and multiple drug interactions.
- Bupropion (Wellbutrin), an antidepressant, has been tried with an inconsistent effect, as some patients improved and some worsened.
- Riluzole (Rilutek) is a drug approved for the treatment of multiple sclerosis. There are some reports of its usefulness in OCD.

Again, these drugs are not approved for OCD. There is little data to support their use (alone or with SSRIs), especially in children. Each has particular side effects and risks, and some are quite dangerous and illegal (e.g., hallucinogens). Any unapproved therapy outside of a **clinical trial** should be carefully considered and fully discussed with your child's physician before trying.

As many as 40% of those treated with one anti-OCD medication will have **residual symptoms**. If they are severe and do not respond to CBT, drug augmentation will be necessary. In children, there has been little to no research done, and what is used is based on what is known about the treatment of resistant OCD in adults.

It is important to be aware that combining medications of any kind, including over-the counter ones, may complicate the treatment of OCD. All the physicians involved in your child's care should be made aware of all medications he or she is taking (including asthma medicines, antibiotics, over-the-counter cough medicines, anti-acne medications, and all others).

Clinical trial

A carefully monitored study of a drug or a treatment using a drug that involves a large group of people with the goal of testing that drug's effectiveness and safety.

Residual symptoms

Symptoms that persist even when treatment has been received at a good therapeutic dose and for the usual length of time usually needed.

77. The doctor wants to give my daughter with OCD a drug used for psychotic patients. But she is not psychotic and knows what is real and what is not. Why do they want to use an antipsychotic drug?

Antipsychotic medications are used mostly to increase the effectiveness of the SSRI medications used in OCD when the results with these medications are small or incomplete. Studies have shown that the use of a second drug as an "augmentation agent" can be more effective than using the SSRI alone.

In some case reports, SSRIs have been augmented with a low dose of risperidone (Risperdal). Currently, only two second-generation antipsychotics have been approved by the FDA for use in children: risperidone (Risperdal) and aripiprazole (Abilify).

The FDA has not approved these drugs for use in OCD; thus, their use in OCD is experimental. The reasons for this lack of approval are varied. Sometimes there has not been enough research done (particularly in children) by the drug companies to convince the FDA to approve the drug. Sometimes no research has been done at all. Other times the research showed the drugs did not work, or the research was inconclusive.

However, many physicians use drugs approved by the FDA for one disease in another disease for which the drug is not approved, particularly when all of the approved therapies have failed. If such a drug is proposed for your child, you should discuss very frankly with your child's physician the reasons why he or she wants to use this drug, what his or her experience with the proposed drug has been, what the possible benefits and risks are, and what special precautions must be taken. You may want to consider a second opinion.

Studies have shown that the use of a second drug as an "augmentation agent" can be more effective than using the SSRI alone.

78. What if we can't afford the medications? Is there any way to get help?

Yes, there is help. Many of the companies that manufacture the medications have assistance programs to provide either a discount or free medications for patients who cannot afford them. The first place to look is the Pharmaceutical Research and Manufacturers Association (PhRMA), which supports many of these special programs and has a Web site where you can check for further information: The Partnership for Prescription Assistance (http://www.pparx.org/Intro.php). They also publish a directory of programs for those who cannot afford the medicines. Your doctor can request this by calling 202-835-3450.

In addition, the pharmaceutical companies can be contacted directly:

- Luvox: Jazz Pharmaceuticals
  650-496-3777; http://www.jazzpharma.com
- Prozac: Lilly Cares Foundation Patient Assistance Program
  800-545-6962 or 800-488-2133; http://www.lilly.com/products/access/direct_patient.html
- Zoloft: Pfizer Inc.
  1-866-776-3700; http://www.pfizerhelpfulanswers.com/pages/Find/findresult.aspx
- Anafranil: Novartis Patient Assistance Program
  1-800-277-2254; http://www.pharma.us.novartis.com/about-us/our-patient-caregiver-resources

See also the excellent listing of such programs at Mental Health Today (www.mental-health-today.com/medsassist.htm).

Parents of 11-year-old Jamal said:

We had a lot of trouble at home and at school with Jamal, who is 11 years old. He's a good kid but was not doing well in school, and he wouldn't tell us why. But the teacher told us he did not pay a lot of attention and was always arranging things on his desk. He also seemed to be bullied a lot, which Jamal never told us about. He also never got around to finishing his homework because he was busy with other things in his room, which we didn't see because he kept the door closed. Finally, when it looked like he might be left back last year in school, we had him evaluated by our pediatrician who thought there might be an emotional problem but was not sure and referred us to a child psychiatrist at the medical center. The psychiatrist spoke with Jamal and with us several times over about 10 days and said that Jamal had moderate OCD. We were shocked and upset, but the psychiatrist told us that it was treatable and recommended both behavioral therapy (which, luckily they did at the medical center) as well as an SSRI. Although the appointments are difficult (and expensive) because we have to take time off from work, Jamal is now a B+ student at school, and the teacher tells us that the bullying seems to have stopped (the school took some measures of its own on this too). His symptoms have markedly decreased. He's not quite an angel, but life at home is now much more pleasant. It took about 2 or 3 months before we saw any improvement, and that was discouraging. But we kept at it and it paid off. The doctor says we may even see more improvement over the next few months. She will decide about possibly decreasing the therapy and the SSRI in several months.

79. Our daughter's psychiatrist thinks she has another psychiatric disorder in addition to the OCD. What other conditions could she have, and how does this affect the treatment?

Many other diseases may be seen in junction with OCD. Unfortunately, having OCD does not prevent or protect someone from having another disorder. Some of these conditions and their treatments include:

Tourette syndrome: This disorder can be treated with SRIs; adding an antipsychotic drug might benefit the two disorders.

Chronic motor tics without Tourette syndrome: This disorder may respond better to clomipramine than SSRIs. Tics may respond to the addition of an antipsychotic drug.

Major depression: Treating the depression is critical. In severe depression with suicidal thoughts, hospitalization is necessary for safety. Comorbid depression does not change the response of OCD symptoms to the SSRIs. Severe depression interferes with the practice of CBT; in those cases, it is necessary to treat the depression before or during a trial of CBT.

Bipolar disorder: Mood stabilization is necessary before starting treatment with an antidepressant drug because antidepressants may induce or increase mania. Bipolar children will need to be treated usually with multiple medicines that may include lithium, anticonvulsants, and antipsychotic drugs. It is only when the bipolar disorder is under control that OCD symptoms will be treated. Risk for suicide needs to be evaluated. Drug interactions must be considered.

Panic disorder: Medicines need to be started at low doses and be increased slowly. Benzodiazepines may be used at the beginning of the treatment for a short period of time to decrease the anxiety.

Social phobia: This disorder responds well to SRIs. MAOIs are effective, but they cannot be combined with SRIs. They have multiple risks and are very rarely used in children and adolescents.

Schizophrenia: These children have abnormalities in the perception or expression of reality, most commonly manifesting as auditory **hallucinations**, paranoid or bizarre delusions, or disorganized speech and thinking in the context of significant social or occupational dysfunction. Some antipsychotic drugs like clozapine

---

Social phobia

A marked and persistent fear of one or more social or performance situations, exposure to unfamiliar people, or to possible scrutiny by others. The person fears acting in an anxious way that will be embarrassing or humiliating.

Hallucination

The apparent, often strong subjective perception of an object or event when no such stimulus or situation is present; may be visual, auditory, tactile, or involve smell or taste sensations.

(Clozaril) might worsen the OCD symptoms. Olanzapine (Zyprexa) monotherapy may be helpful. Adding
fluvoxamine (Luvox) to control the OCD symptoms
may work. CBT may be tried.

Substance use disorders: These disorders can cause poor
adherence to OCD treatment as well as drug interactions. Treating these disorders before or during OCD
treatment is necessary.

Autism and Asperger syndrome: Repetitive thoughts and
behaviors are frequent in autism and Asperger syndrome. SRIs and CBT can be used.

Neurological conditions: These conditions are treated
before the OCD, when possible.

80. How do you know when the acute phase of OCD is over? When does the maintenance treatment start, and what is done?

The acute phase is over in your child when you, your child,
and the treatment team agree that the symptoms are minimal
and that the disruption and turbulence at home or at school
is over. There is no absolute definition for this; it may actually occur gradually before you realize one day that home and
school life has become much calmer and easier. At this point,
maintenance becomes the main goal. The treatment gains that
have been achieved need to be maintained.

First, when the treatment is successful, a new schedule for
visits to the therapist needs to be set up. Often this schedule
consists of monthly follow-up visits for at least 6 months and
then less frequently if your child is staying on maintenance
therapy that is not being changed.

Next, your child's physician at some point may want to consider decreasing or stopping the treatment. He or she will

discuss this with you and your child, and a plan will be developed. This adjustment may require that doctor visits remain fairly frequent to be sure that relapses do not occur.

Some general comments about maintenance therapy:

Children who have not received CBT in addition to medication have a higher risk of relapse.

- Children who have not received CBT in addition to medication have a higher risk of relapse. It is recommended that they continue the medicine longer.
- OCD is a chronic condition, and OCD medications are not a cure. Your child may need to take the medicine indefinitely. Sometimes, when the medication is withdrawn, the OCD symptoms return to their pre-drug level of severity.
- Some children or adolescents may need lifelong **prophylactic** treatment after two to four severe relapses or three to four mild relapses.
- No one knows exactly how long patients should take these medications once they have been effective. Some children are able to discontinue them after 6 to 12 months of treatment. Some physicians say that the treatment should continue for at least 1 year. There is no consensus on this point, so it is largely one of trial and error with the goal of minimizing or ending the medication so long as symptoms are minimal to none.
- If the maintenance treatment has been successful, the therapist will often propose trying to discontinue the medication(s) but in a very gradual manner. One regimen uses a lowering of the dose by 25% every 2 months if it is well tolerated, while giving CBT booster sessions. It seems that the risk of relapse is lower if children learn to use behavioral therapy techniques while they are doing well on the medications. The behavioral techniques may help the patients to control any symptoms that might return when they stop the medications.
- If discontinuation of treatment is planned (particularly if it should occur during summer vacation), the parents and the child should be prepared for a potential relapse

Prophylactic

Prevention of a disease or process that can lead to a disease.

and educated about the need to reinstitute the treatment at the earliest sign of relapse. After medications are stopped, symptoms usually do not return immediately. They may take a few weeks to months before being seen.

- There is a small risk that should a child relapse after discontinuation, reinstitution of the previously effective medication may produce poorer results this time. This risk needs to be taken into account when deciding whether to stop drug therapy.
- And finally, as noted previously, abrupt withdrawal of the SSRI may be associated with a withdrawal syndrome—another reason for a slow tapering of any medication.

Nancy's father said:

We had a really tough time with Nancy (who is now 9). She developed bad symptoms when she was 7 with lots of rituals and obsessions—particularly about germs and cleanliness. Our washing machine bills were sky high, as she made us wash her clothes separately from the rest of the family's. At first we thought it was just a quirk or something, but it was getting out of hand, so we had her evaluated by a psychologist and then a child psychiatrist. They said she had a fairly severe case of OCD but were hopeful that treatment would really reduce her symptoms. She started right away on an SSRI, but it did not work at all. We kept it up for 6 months (probably too long when I look back now) and then the doctor switched to a different one. Finally we started to see some decrease in symptoms, though it required two dosage increases. Nancy had some mild side effects when the dose was raised each time, but they went away quickly. Although both the doctor and psychologist wanted to do behavioral therapy, we could not afford this, unfortunately (our health plan did not cover it). But we're glad the medicine is helping. She is acting better, and her germ and cleanliness obsessions really only appear when she is stressed at school (like with big science tests).

81. When should we consider hospitalization for our child? Or an intensive OCD residential treatment center?

Children or adolescents may need to be hospitalized in a psychiatric unit if they are a danger to others or to themselves (i.e., presenting a risk of suicide or self-injurious behaviors), or if their level of impairment is very severe and is harming their development.

Some situations in which hospitalization should be considered include:

- If your child has multiple other diseases that will need to be treated at the same time as the OCD
- If your child did not tolerate previous treatments well
- If your child is an adolescent and is using drugs (in which case, his or her compliance with treatment might be so poor that the only safe place to receive treatment might be an inpatient unit)
- If the family stressors are so high that removing the child from the home for a period of time is the only solution
- If your child is exposed to any abuse, physical or sexual (hospitalization might be a temporary safe place until the situation is resolved)

Hospitalization may be prolonged if your child is not ready to return home and needs further and more structured treatment that absolutely cannot be done at home.

Another possibility is intensive treatment programs. They are usually residential centers that are highly specialized in treating OCD. They can be used when all usual treatments have been tried and nothing seems to be working. Decisions about residential placement are usually made by the family, the treatment team, and sometimes the school team. These programs can be contacted by you or your child's psychiatrist.

The current list is available through the Obsessive Compulsive Foundation (http://www.ocfoundation.org/ocd-intensive-treatment-programs.html).

82. Should I place my child with OCD in a clinical research treatment trial for a new drug?

This question is both philosophical and very personal for your family. On the societal level, progress with new techniques and medications will not occur without clinical testing. Participating in this testing, however, means exposing your child to a therapy for which there is little experience; the therapy may or may not work, and it may or may not have side effects. Therefore, while you may be motivated to help with the development of new treatment techniques, this is your child, and the decision will have a large impact on your child and your family.

Participating in this testing means exposing your child to a therapy for which there is little experience; the therapy may or may not work, and it may or may not have side effects.

There is no correct answer to this question. If you seek such experimental therapies or if they are proposed to you, it is your obligation to fully inform yourself of the data known already and to get an understanding of the known potential risks and benefits. Remember that you must by law be fully informed and enter into the trial freely and without coercion. Your child (or you, if your child is not old enough legally to sign in your jurisdiction) will be asked to sign an informed consent. There is a patient's "bill of rights" that you should examine, and you will be informed who to contact for questions, issues, and emergencies. You have the right to withdraw from the trial at any time for any (or no) reason at all without prejudicing future care—that is, you will not be "punished" for leaving the trial.

Research participants are frequently sought locally or nationally. Usually the treatments are done in academic or regional centers that organize the trials, and all treatments are free. Travel expenses may be reimbursed.

However, it is a commitment on your part to follow the trial's treatment protocol. You and your child's physician may review the clinical trials underway and discuss whether your child might benefit from one of them. Ultimately, the clinical investigator at the trial site will decide if your child meets the inclusion and exclusion criteria for the trial and if the trial can accept him or her.

In considering this decision, you should take multiple factors into account, including:

- How well your child is doing on his or her current therapy
- What the trial is proposing in terms of drugs or other therapy
- Whether the proposed treatment is added on to the current treatment or replaces it
- Whether there is a washout period (no treatment during this time)
- The duration of the trial
- What will happen when the trial ends (that is, if the new drug has worked, will you be able to continue it "off protocol" under a compassionate use program)
- If two different treatments or drugs are offered, which one your child will get

You can look for clinical trial information on the Obsessive Compulsive Foundation Web site (http://www.ocfoundation. org/research-participants-sought.html) and at the world-wide registry Web site run by the U.S. National Institutes of Health (http://clinicaltrials.gov/ct2/home).

83. What about alternative and natural remedies? Would prayer work?

You will see on the Internet and in publications lots of claims for new, different, natural, organic, or other remedies. Other than what is noted in this book, no treatments that have been rigorously tested in a scientific manner have been consistently shown to work in treating OCD.

Single reports or cases of success or anecdotes claiming that a particular treatment works in a patient are very common in medicine. The problem here is that a disease like OCD that waxes and wanes may improve (or worsen) on its own, whether the proposed treatment was given or not. Also, remember that few people will publish reports or cases of their failures; rather, they only publish successful reports. In clinical medicine, the gold standard for new treatments is to do clinical trials using the new treatment in one group of children and the older or standard treatment in the other group; or, both groups receive the standard treatment and one of the groups receives the new treatment in addition. Only by comparing treatments in a sufficient number of patients can one make claims of effectiveness. The FDA requires such testing of new drugs before approving them for use in the United States.

Be very wary of anything that claims total or 100% success, any medical therapy that uses the word "miracle," and any suggestions that the proposed therapy has been suppressed by the established medical system. These claims should all be received with great suspicion.

Whether prayer works is in part a philosophical and religious question that is certainly beyond the scope of this book. However, there is a large medical literature supporting positive attitude and the desire to be made well as benefits to treatment. There is an interesting Web site that reviews some of the information on OCD and religion from the Christian, Jewish, and Islamic points of view (www.geonius.com/ocd/religion.html#Judaism).

84. I heard that new therapies are in progress for treatment–resistant OCD? Can we expect anything new and better soon?

Several lines of research are underway both with medications and other modalities of treatment for OCD. However, nothing has yet clearly shown treatment advances, and these experimental methods are only being done in a few centers around the country, usually for patients with very severe forms of OCD. Most of this work is in adult patients, not children.

Transcranial magnetic stimulation (repetitive TMS, rTMS): In this treatment, magnetic pulses are focused on a part of the brain called the supplementary motor area (SMA), which plays a role in filtering out internal stimuli such as ruminations, obsessions, and tics. The TMS treatment is an attempt to normalize the SMA's activity so that it properly filters out thoughts and behaviors associated with OCD. Its advantages are that it is non-invasive (e.g., no needles, shocks) and well tolerated. However, it must be given daily, and there are often mild headaches after stimulation.

Electroconvulsive therapy (electroshock, ECT): This treatment involves electrically stimulating the brain under anesthesia. It is not as widely used today as it was in the past. Its primary use is in very severe depression unresponsive to other treatments. It is also used in bipolar disorders. For OCD, there is possible efficacy but no standard treatment. There are risks and side effects, including memory loss, and it is reserved for treatment-resistant OCD with co-occurring conditions, such as life-threatening major depression.

Deep brain stimulation: This technique involves the surgical implantation in the brain of a so-called brain pacemaker. This device sends electrical charges to parts of the brain. It has been used to treat depression, Parkinson disease, tremor, and chronic pain. The advantages of the procedure include its reversibility in comparison to other neurosurgery techniques. Beneficial effects appeared over variable times, ranging from 3 weeks to several months. Disadvantages include that it is an invasive procedure with the risk of brain hemorrhage, infections, and seizures. Side effects include fatigue, memory disturbances, tingling, nausea, and diarrhea.

Neurosurgical stereotactic lesion procedures: This term includes various neurosurgery techniques (also performed via radiosurgery, known as "gamma-knife" procedures) to cut out or cut certain parts of the brain. Unlike the brain pacemaker, these techniques are irreversible. They are all highly selective treatments performed for very few patients with the most severe cases of OCD. Complications have been seen and vary with the parts of the brain that have been treated. Seizures and hallucinations have been described in bilateral anterior capsulotomy. Memory disturbances, apathy, urinary disturbances, seizures, and hydrocephalus were seen with multiple cingulotomies. Headaches, low grade fever, nausea, vomiting, somnolence, and apathy were seen in limbic leucotomy. These procedures are reserved for only the most extremely severe, refractory cases, and these techniques should only be done in centers with experience doing them.

Chang's mother said:

We are having real issues with our 8-year-old son Chang. He was diagnosed with OCD last year by a child psychiatrist in our town and was started on an SSRI and behavioral therapy. It really didn't help much, unfortunately. The doctor switched to a different SSRI and tried raising the dose twice, but it didn't do much, and the side effects were worse. He tried a third one and then added another drug for augmentation. There was some very mild improvement, but the compulsions continued (especially list making—he goes through 5 spiral notebooks a month making color-coded lists). We know the doctor has tried pretty much everything. He just suggested that we go to the medical school in the city about 75 miles away where they seem to be doing research and using experimental techniques. We're going to do that, though we're a bit afraid of using experimental things on our son. But we don't know what more we can do.

PART SIX

The Family, School, and Siblings

Should I try to get the rest of the family to help in the treatment of my child? What should I tell them?

Should I tell my daughter's school that she has OCD? Whom do I tell, and how do I do this?

Help! My health insurance carrier has very limited reimbursement for OCD treatment and support functions. What can I do?

More . . .

85. Should I try to get the rest of the family to help in the treatment of my child? What should I tell them?

Yes, most definitely. Family involvement and support is crucial. The family needs to work as a team in the fight against OCD. Education of all family members is necessary as well as acceptance of the child as he or she is. With education, your family can help maintain the structure and discipline that are so important in preventing your child's OCD from unnecessarily disrupting family life.

Structure

All children need structure and a daily routine that makes them feel secure. Nobody likes change, least of all a child with OCD.

All children need structure and a daily routine that makes them feel secure. OCD symptoms are more severe when there are life changes. Set clear rules and expectations for the child. Give the rules in a positive way; for example, you may say, "Do your homework before watching TV," instead of, "No TV until your homework is done." Structure and schedule activities for each day. Have family dinner, homework, and bedtime at the same time most days. If a change happens, help your child to accept it. Nobody likes change, least of all a child with OCD .

Discipline

Misbehavior occurs and frequently has nothing to do with the OCD. Set up a behavioral program for the child and reward good behavior. The rewards (and punishments) will depend on the age, temperament, and personality of each child. Have the child decide on which behavior he wants to work on. Give small rewards, such as points or stickers (not big or expensive items). Praise is a fine reward in many circumstances along with a little treat (such as some "quality time," playing a game together, reading a special book, a special snack, or a token for a movie). Do not let the child with OCD avoid taking responsibility for negative behavior that he or she can control.

Tell your family members that OCD is not fair! It is not fair for the child with the disease, and it is not fair for the family, in particular the brothers and the sisters. They may feel that their sibling gets away with things because of the OCD, and they are probably correct at times. Education about the disease and treatment will help them to understand and to not blame the child with OCD or you, the parent.

It is also hard to explain why one child has OCD and not the others. You should explain that there are interactions between genetics, biology, and environment that probably made this happen. Reassuring the other children that they will not catch the OCD is important.

86. Should I tell my daughter's school that she has OCD? Whom do I tell, and how do I do this?

Yes. A child's teacher, the school counselor, and the school nurse are important team members in the fight against OCD. They sometimes may not know much about OCD and may need to be gently taught. Your daughter may have tried very hard to hide her symptoms from her school friends or teachers, complicating matters.

Nonetheless, the teacher may observe:

- A decline in academic performance
- Messy homework with a lot of erased spots or holes in the papers
- Unfinished homework
- Falling asleep in class
- Asking to go to the bathroom frequently and spending a lot of time there
- Misbehavior done purposely to camouflage compulsive behaviors
- Daydreaming and lack of attention during class
- Depression and isolation from the other children

The Family, School, and Siblings

You need to communicate to the teacher what is happening and give information about the disease if needed. The teacher and the school nurse need to know if your daughter takes medications and what the possible side effects are. Special management or accommodations may be needed in the classroom, at recess, and at lunchtime. You should also communicate the progress of behavioral therapy. Your daughter's teacher will be able to discuss her school behavior and progress with you—and, with your consent, possibly with her therapist.

87. My child seems to be teased by the other kids and has lost his friends. Is it due to his OCD?

When the OCD is severe and visible, your child may indeed get teased or ridiculed. Peer victimization is frequent among children with OCD. Your son's self-esteem will be negatively affected, as the OCD often leads to embarrassing situations. It can affect friendships because of the amount of time wasted on the rituals and not having enough time to play with friends. Children are often not the most tolerant of people and may react negatively to unusual OCD-related behaviors. They may call your son names like "crazy"—or worse. Children with OCD may try to hide their symptoms with variable success. Feelings of loneliness, depression, and anger may follow when their social life suffers.

Children with OCD may try to hide their symptoms with variable success. Feelings of loneliness, depression, and anger may follow when their social life suffers.

When teasing occurs, it is necessary to rapidly address the situation. You should approach your son's teacher, counselor, and others in the school as necessary to discuss ways to rectify the situation. Schools are becoming more and more aware of bullying and other such negative behavior, and should have techniques and methods to address this situation.

Social difficulty is one reason why it is so important to recognize the disease early on and to become well educated about it as a family. Timely recognition will lead to a medical/psychiatric evaluation early in the game and to the best individualized treatment. It is only then that your family will be able to help your son cope with the illness and its complications, at home and at school.

Speak with your son's therapist to discuss his social difficulties. It might be possible to integrate your son into group therapy to improve his social skills and self-esteem.

88. We can live with our son's OCD except for homework time, which is a nightmare. What can we do?

Homework time can be very frustrating. Here are a few things you can do to help:

- Know if your son is returning his assignments and how long he spends on his homework. If it is too much at a certain time, discuss it with his teacher.
- Provide a special and comfortable place away from his siblings where he can do his homework and where all needed supplies are readily available.
- Schedule homework time at the same time each day after quiet activities. Make sure that the activities your son is involved in before starting his homework can be easily finished so that he does not start his homework frustrated and unhappy.
- Arrange to have homework time everyday at the same time, even if there is no homework given that day by the teacher. This time should be at least 30 minutes long and should involve another kind of learning activity if there is no homework that day.
- Help your son to break any large task into smaller tasks. What seems insurmountable as a whole can be readily handled if it is cut into multiple small tasks.
- Make sure your son takes breaks between tasks without getting involved in another big chore or activity. Hard though it may be, try to arrange it so he has a little fun doing homework.

- Reward your son with praise and/or stickers (or some other small item) when he has completed the homework without temper tantrums or whining.

As previously noted, communicate with your child's teacher through visits, phone calls, and notes, as decided early in the term.

89. My daughter with OCD is very bright, but her grades and academic performance are bad? Why is this? What should I do?

Intellectual functioning is not impaired in OCD. Most people with OCD have normal intelligence. Some children with mental retardation or with pervasive developmental disorders (such as autism or Asperger syndrome) may have repetitive behaviors, rituals, and symptoms of OCD with obsessions and compulsions, but these conditions are different than OCD by itself.

Low academic performance may be due to a number of causes, some of which may be related to OCD (see Question 86) and some not. You should work with your daughter's psychiatrist and the school team to determine the causes of her low grades and how to address this problem. If the issue turns out to be OCD symptoms interfering with academic functioning, you should discuss this with your child's psychiatrist. If it turns out to be something else, this probably is best handled with the teacher and school team. In many cases it may be a combination of the two requiring some assistance from both the medical and school teams.

90. I found out that my son's school has not been responsive to his needs, and he may have to repeat his grade. What should I do?

If the situation has reached this point, with the support of your child psychiatrist, you will need to contact the school, as it may be time to ask for a child study team evaluation.

After this request, in most jurisdictions, the school has a certain amount of time to provide the evaluation (it is usually about 90 days). As part of the evaluation, your son will undergo a psychiatric evaluation (usually the school will accept one done by your child psychiatrist), a psychological evaluation, a learning evaluation, and a **psychosocial** evaluation done by a school social worker. If your son needs something more, such as a neurological evaluation or a speech and hearing evaluation, it can be offered as well.

Psychosocial

The impact of social situations and mental health upon each other.

The child study team will review the results and make a recommendation in writing called an Individualized Education Plan (IEP). You will be asked to review this plan in the school at a special meeting. You should discuss the report with your son's therapist, who should also receive a copy.

You should try to make an objective determination as to whether the school's position is in fact correct for your son. If you are not satisfied, however, you may appeal. In some cases, you may need a professional educational advocate to assist you in this process. At the extreme, the legal system may have to be involved.

12-year-old Cindy said:

I have a lot of problems in school. I cannot pay attention because I am always worried about everything. Sometimes I think my mom is going to die in a car accident or that I may stab her. I put away all sharp objects from my room and my desk. If these thoughts come at school, I need to touch something from right to left and tap it a certain amount of times (sometimes 6 times, sometimes 10 times). The tapping has to make some noise, and if it does not, I need to do it again. Kids in my class think I am a freak. Sometimes, I think I am one too. Writing is a problem because I get upset if some of the letters are not completely closed, like an "a" or an "o," and I go over them to make sure that they are. Some letters cannot be touched by others. If they are, I have to erase them and rewrite them. My teacher says that my work is messy. I never have enough time to finish my work. I am trying hard, but I will have to repeat my grade this year.

The Family, School, and Siblings

91. We tried a behavioral program and our daughter's OCD actually got worse. We gave up. Any suggestions?

You should remember that things usually get worse before they get better. Children (and adults) do not usually like change. For example, if you stop offering reassurance to your daughter or doing what she asks of you after having done it regularly for a long period of time, she is going to press you by asking more frequently or more aggressively for the reassurance that is now gone. She may become very angry at you. However, once she learns that she will not get the desired response, she will eventually stop asking. (This phenomenon is called "extinction.")

It may be extremely difficult to get her to engage in the treatment—she may even refuse to participate. Do not give up hope. A good working relationship with the therapist will help your child make progressive changes and improvements. But it may take some time. Be patient.

Do not make it easier for your daughter to live with her OCD. Being uncomfortable with the symptoms may motivate her to change.

Do not make it easier for your daughter to live with her OCD. Being uncomfortable with the symptoms may motivate her to change. There is a vicious cycle in OCD, as rituals feed the cycle. You may realize that you have actually fed the cycle by enabling the rituals or by saying unhelpful things (usually with good intentions to diminish her suffering). An example might be washing clothes repeatedly when your child asks, even though the clothes are clean. The next time she becomes fearful of their uncleanliness, the cycle will restart and she will ask you to wash them again. If you do it, it will decrease your daughter's anxiety, but it will reinforce the vicious cycle.

Do things step by step. You cannot change everything at once. Pick one action that enables your child to continue her ritual and work on changing that. For example, work on the rewashing of clean clothes. Explain to your child what you are going to change in your own behavior and why. Be very consistent. You need to follow through with what you said you will change, and you need to do this all the time. Say what you'll do, and do what you say. Involve the other family members as well so your child will not be able to turn to them to gratify her requests by playing them against you.

Be supportive of your daughter as she is going to have added anxiety during this period. And be ready for a possible difficult ride.

Do not forget to look after yourself and to satisfy your own needs, which are different from your child's. Take time for yourself.

92. Is my son going to be called "crazy" because he has OCD? I don't want him to be stigmatized for the rest of his life. Should I refuse treatment and allow him to get better on his own ?

A person is not "crazy" for having a mental illness. OCD is a malfunction in the brain due to organic causes and can be treated. Taking medication is not a stigma these days. A lot of people, including young children, take medications for different reasons.

Nevertheless, medications should be given to children (and adults) only when it is absolutely necessary. It is only if the child is in much distress that they should be given. However, to not use them when the situation is severe and the treating physician thinks they will help would be truly unfair to your son, as his development will continue to be impaired by the untreated disease and his emotional state will continue to be unstable.

Non-drug treatment using CBT only would be ideal. However, in many cases, CBT does not give full relief to the child or is unavailable. You should use all known treatments that are potentially helpful and available. This decision is to be made by the family, the doctor, and your son. You have to work as a team for the long-term benefit of your child.

93. My daughter's pediatrician says her symptoms will disappear if we wait, but the psychiatrist doesn't agree. Should we wait or should we be aggressive in starting treatment?

Very mild symptoms usually do not require treatment. However, you may not be aware of the full extent of your child's symptoms, either because she has learned to hide them or disguise them from you or because they are primarily mental compulsions (like counting or repeating words in her head) that you do not see. It is largely up to your child's doctors to determine if the level of OCD should or should not be treated at this point. If there is disagreement, you may want to suggest that the two physicians speak with each other to come to an agreement.

There should be regular and periodic reevaluation to see if anything is changing as your daughter develops. There is also a tendency by parents to minimize their children's problems. The majority of kids with OCD usually do not grow out of it. Results from research studies show a wide range (10 to 50%) of children having a complete remission by late adolescence. Most children have some symptoms that they will be able to manage with treatment.

If your daughter's symptoms are very infrequent, do not distress her or anyone in the family, and do not impair her functioning at home, school, or with friends, then it seems you can wait. But as soon as she becomes unhappy about the symptoms, her academic functioning suffers, or her relationships become tense, consider the treatment option. Do not hesitate to have a child psychiatrist evaluate your child, as OCD is frequently undiagnosed or misdiagnosed and has frequent delays in its treatment. Many pediatricians do not have much experience in diagnosing or treating OCD. Treating it early can reduce the severity of the symptoms, enhance normal growth and development, and improve your daughter's quality of life.

94. My child is refusing to go to school because of his rituals. What can I do?

It is not uncommon for a young, distressed, anxious child with OCD to refuse to go to school. Children with OCD are caught in behaviors that they cannot stop and that make them feel very unhappy. They may be ashamed in front of their teachers and peers. They may be ridiculed and bullied by their classmates. They may not be able to finish their homework on time. They may get easily frustrated and angry. Their self-esteem may suffer.

Sometimes these children would rather be punished for not going to school than have to face the difficulties waiting for them there. They may become depressed and withdrawn or regressed, wanting to stay home with a parent who frequently enables them to continue their rituals with little objection, which makes them feel better. Also, children with OCD may have other anxiety disorders, like panic attacks, generalized anxiety, or **separation anxiety** that will need to be diagnosed and treated.

95. My son seems to feel guilty and blames himself for the bad thoughts he has. Should we tell him they are not his fault? Actually, are they his fault?

Teach your son what OCD is. OCD is not his fault. The bad thoughts and worries are not who he is. They are a part of the OCD (disease) and are independent of him. Keep in mind:

- OCD symptoms are independent of the child's volition or choice. They cannot be controlled by the child, who really does not want to have them.
- Children who have bad thoughts (particularly young children) think they themselves are bad and will frequently hide the thoughts from their parents. It is important that the parents understand what is occurring by communicating honestly with their child to try

Children with OCD are caught in behaviors that they cannot stop and that make them feel very unhappy. They may be ashamed in front of their teachers and peers.

Separation anxiety

A psychological condition in which an individual has excessive anxiety regarding separation from home or from people to whom the individual has a strong emotional attachment (like a father and mother).

The Family, School, and Siblings

121

to draw out his or her fears and problems in a supportive and non-threatening way.

- Children, when they understand that OCD is a disease
  and is not their fault, will do much better.
- Group therapy will help your child to see that he or she
  is not alone in having problems. If you cannot find an
  OCD group in your area, another group may be useful
  (e.g., coping skills, anger management, social group).
  (See Questions 55 and 56)
- For a younger child, to give the OCD a name like Mr.
  Worry or Mr. Clean may help the child to differentiate
  the disease from himself or herself.

96. I disagree with my husband about giving medications to our child for her OCD. What should we do?

You and your spouse must be united to help your child. Go
together to discuss the issue with your child's psychiatrist,
who will be able to explain why medication has been recommended. During this meeting, both of you will be able to
discuss all the concerns you have. If there are misconceptions
about the treatment or misunderstandings, the doctor may be
able to correct or clarify them. He or she will be able to educate both of you on the disease and treatment alternatives.

If you still disagree about the treatment, the doctor will try
to find alternatives. Some children may be started only on
cognitive-behavioral therapy in which both of you will be
involved and a time limit will be created to review the results.
If further or different treatment is needed later on, a review
of the benefits and risks of each treatment can be done at the
doctor's office, and a change in the direction of treatment may
then be better accepted.

97. I am a single mother and everything falls on me. I am overwhelmed and at the end of my rope. What can I do?

It is extremely difficult to deal with this situation by yourself. You may feel helpless and very sad to see your child struggling with the illness. But in fact, you are not alone. You can have a very supportive team of therapists working with you (the doctor, the psychologist or social worker, and the school staff). Perhaps your friends or family can offer support (e.g., grandparents, uncles, aunts).

You may ask the doctor (and insurance company, if required) if a behavioral therapist could come to your home on a regular basis to help you organize a treatment plan in your own environment. There are case management agencies that can help you for additional services. You can go to a parent support group if one is available in your area. The Obsessive Compulsive Foundation is a wonderful reference to call or to visit online (http://www.ocfoundation.org). Chat rooms on the Internet dedicated to parents of children with OCD may be useful also (try searching for "OCD chat room").

98. In the area where I live, there is no behavioral therapist. What should I do?

It might be worth considering going to an out-of-area therapist, if this is feasible, on a less frequent basis.

Alternatively, *you* can become your child's therapist, but you will need to be well prepared. You can find information on the Internet, or you can go to your local library and read about the behavioral treatment. There are also a lot of books available adapted in a very practical way to the cognitive-behavioral treatment of children. Choose one or two that fit your child's developmental age.

> You *can become your child's therapist, but you will need to be well prepared.*

After going through the material, define exactly which symptom (for example, hand washing) you intend to eliminate. Start with only one symptom at a time. Put in place a clear plan that you explain to your child. Start by working on preventing the ritual. Although this will initially produce some anxiety, if done gently, the level of anxiety should be tolerable. Be consistent in practicing every day with your child, and progressively increase the difficulty of the task (for example, by increasing the time until the ritual can be completed—hand washing in this example). Be firm and supportive with your child. Be positive; praise any success or, at the beginning, even just the attempts.

You should review your plan with your child's psychiatrist.

99. I work full time, and my child is in school. It is hard to schedule all the appointments. Do we have to miss school and work for treatment?

In the current work environment, many employers are now aware of and sympathetic to family issues that parents must deal with. A parent may need to miss work to get medical care for a child. Speak with your employer or your human resources department for help. Be prepared to offer your employer compensation for their assistance. For example, if you need to miss 3 hours for an appointment once a month, offer to work an hour more for the next 3 days to make up the time. Or offer to do the missed work at home if that is possible. If both parents are available, try to alternate the visits between the two of you so that neither one loses all the time. Employers do not want to have to replace workers who are serious, productive, and helpful to their business. Most will try to work things out.

See if there is any way to schedule appointments early or late in the day to minimize time lost. This may require scheduling the appointments well in advance.

Your child's OCD may worsen if untreated. It also may interfere significantly with his or her education and development.
So it makes sense to miss school sometimes for the appointments. Schools also are more flexible in many respects now
than they were in the past. Speak with your child's teacher
and principal if needed. If you show yourself to be caring and
desirous of working out a solution that is a win-win for all
concerned, you will usually see a lot of flexibility on the part
of the school. Try to avoid confrontation, but strive to work
things out.

100. Help! My health insurance carrier has very limited reimbursement for OCD treatment and support functions. What can I do?

This is a major problem in the United States. Many mental
health functions are not reimbursed or are reimbursed at a
level below that of a "medical" disease (like asthma). You will
need to make use of the appeal and preapproval mechanisms
that most insurance companies have in place. You may need
to involve your doctor and the hospital or clinic administrator
or social worker to assist in the appeal process. As noted in
Question 78 , there are programs for lower cost or even free
medication determined on a need basis. You may be able to
find less expensive assistance at county or other governmental
clinics or in medical schools if nearby.

Appendix

Support Groups

Obsessive Compulsive Foundation (OCF)
Lists a large number of support groups in different locations around the world. For a small membership fee, further information and a bimonthly newsletter are available.
OC Foundation
PO Box 961029
Boston, MA 02196
Phone: (617) 973-5801
Fax: (617) 973-5803
E-mail: http://info@ocfoundation.org
Web site: www.ocfoundation.org

Obsessive Compulsive Information Center (OCIC)
of the Madison Institute of Medicine
OCIC can do computer searches on the latest research and maintains physician referral and support group lists.
Madison Institute of Medicine
7617 Mineral Point Road, Suite 300
Madison, WI 53717
Phone: (608) 827-2470
Fax: (608) 827-2479
Web site: www.miminc.org/aboutocic.asp

Anxiety Disorders Association of America
8730 Georgia Avenue, Suite 600
Silver Spring, MD 20910
Phone: (240) 485-1001
Fax: (240) 485-1035
E-mail: http://information@adaa.org
Web site: www.adaa.org

National Alliance on Mental Illness
Colonial Place Three
2107 Wilson Boulevard, Suite 300
Arlington, VA 22201-3042
Phone: (800) 950-NAMI (Toll Free)
Fax: (703) 524-9094
Web site: www.nami.org

National Institute of Mental Health
Science Writing, Press, and Dissemination Branch
6001 Executive Boulevard, Room 8184, MSC 9663
Bethesda, MD 20892-9663
Phone: (866) 615-6464 (Toll Free)
Fax: (301) 443-4279
E-mail: http://nimhinfo@nih.gov
Web site: www.nimh.nih.gov

Association for Behavioral and Cognitive Therapies
305 7th Avenue, 16th Floor
New York, New York 10001
Phone: (212) 647-1890
Fax: (212) 647-1865
Web site: www.abct.org

Obsessive Compulsive Anonymous
PO Box 215
New Hyde Park, NY 11040
Phone: (516) 739-0662

Freedom From Fear
308 Seaview Avenue
Staten Island, NY 10305
Phone: (718) 351-1717
Fax: (718) 980-5022
E-mail: help@freedomfromfear.org
Web site: http://freedomfromfear.org/

Organizations

American Psychiatric Association (APA)
1000 Wilson Boulevard, Suite 1825
Arlington, VA 22209
Phone: (703) 907-7300
Web site: www.psych.org

Trichotillomania Learning Center
207 McPherson Street, Suite H
Santa Cruz, CA 95060-5863
Phone: (831) 457-1004
Fax: (831) 426-4383
E-mail: http://info@trich.org
Web site: www.trich.org

Tourette Syndrome Association, Inc.
42-45 Bell Boulevard, Suite 205
Bayside, New York 11361-2820
Phone: (718) 224-2999
Web site: www.tsa-usa.org

Learning Disabilities Association of America (LDA)
4156 Library Road
Pittsburg, PA 15234
Phone: (412) 341-1515 or (412) 341-8077
Fax: (412) 344-0224
Web site: www.ldanatl.org

National Dissemination Center for Children with Disabilities (NICHCY)
Provides information about disabilities for families and educators, focusing on children from birth to 22 years of age. It publishes free, fact-filled newsletters and advises about the laws entitling children with disabilities to special education and other services.
NICHCY
PO Box 1492
Washington, DC 20013
Phone: (800) 695-0285
Web site: www.nichcy.org

Federal Resource Center for Special Education
Academy for Educational Development
1825 Connecticut Avenue NW
Washington, DC 20009
Phone: (202) 884-8215
Web site: www.rrfcnetwork.org

Outpatient Clinics Specializing in OCD

Center for the Treatment and Study of Anxiety (University of Pennsylvania, Philadelphia)
www.med.upenn.edu/ctsa

UCLA OCD Day Treatment Program: Intensive Treatment Program (Los Angeles, CA)
www.semel.ucla.edu/adc/

Westwood Institute for Anxiety Disorders: Specializing in OCD (Los Angeles, CA)
http://hope4ocd.com/index.php

Bio-Behavioral Institute: Clinic treating OCD and related disorders (Great Neck, NY)
www.bio-behavioral.com/home.asp

Austin Center for the treatment of OCD (Austin, TX)
http://austinocd.com

NYU Child Study Center (New York City)
www.aboutourkids.org

Inpatient Treatment Centers

McLean OCD Institute (Boston, MA)
www.mclean.harvard.edu/patient/adult/ocd.php

University of Florida Center for the Treatment of OCD (Gainesville, FL)
www.ufocd.org

Menninger Adolescent Treatment Program (Houston, TX)
www.menningerclinic.com/p-ocd/index.htm/p-adolescent/index.htm

Rogers Memorial Hospital (Southeastern Wisconsin)
www.rogershospital.org/obsessive_compulsivedisorders.php

Psychosurgery Centers

Massachusetts General Hospital (Boston, MA)
http://neurosurgery.mgh.harvard.edu/Functional/psysurg.htm

University of Michigan Depression Center
www.depressioncenter.org

Books

For Professionals:

OCD in Children and Adolescents: A Cognitive-Behavioral Treatment Manual by
John S. March and Karen Mulle (Guilford Press,1998)

OCD in Children and Adolescents by Judith L. Rapoport (American Psychiatric
Publishing, Inc, 1988)

*Handbook of Cognitive-Behavior Group Therapy with Children and Adolescents:
Specific Settings and Presenting Problems* by Ray W. Christner, Jessica L.
Stewart, and Arthur Freeman (Routledge, 2007)

Obsessive-Compulsive Disorders: Diagnosis, Etiology, Treatment by Eric Hollander
and Dan J. Stein (Marcel Dekker, 1997)

Overcoming OCD by Gail S. Steketee (New Harbinger, 2008)

For Children:

Up and Down the Worry Hill by Aureen Pinto-Wagner (Lighthouse Press, 2000)

Mr. Worry: A Story About OCD by Holly Niner (Albert Whitman & Company,
2004)

What to Do when Your Brain Gets Stuck: A Kid's Guide to Overcoming OCD by
Dawn Huebner (Magination Press, 2007)

Touch and Go Joe by Joe Wells (Jessica Kingsley Publishers, 2006)

Polly's Magic Games: A Child's View of Obsessive-Compulsive Disorder by
Constance Foster (Dilligaf Publishing, 1994)

Overcoming OCD: A Guide for College Students. Online from Chicago OCD:
www.ocdchicago.org/index.php/college

Blink, Blink, Clop, Clop: Why Do We Do Things We Can't Stop by E. Katia Moritz
(Childswork/Childsplay, 2001)

You Do That Too? by Rena Benson (Dilligaf Publishers, 2000)

Not as Crazy as I Seem by George Harrar (Houghton Mifflin, 2004)

Repetitive Rhonda by Jan Evans (Breath and Shadow Productions, 2007)

A Thought Is Just a Thought: A Story of Living with OCD by Leslie Talley (Lantern Books, 2004)

Kissing Doorknobs by Terry Spencer Hesser (Delacorte Books, 1999)

For Parents:

Family-Based Treatment for Young Children with OCD Workbook by Jennifer B. Freeman and Abbe Marrs Garcia (Oxford University Press, 2008)

Talking Back to OCD: The program That Helps Kids and Teens Say "No Way"—and Parents Say "Way to Go" by John S. March (The Guilford Press, 2006)

The Everything Parent's Guide to Children with OCD: Professional, Reassuring Advice for Raising a Happy, Well-Adjusted Child by Stephen Martin and Victoria Costello (Adams Media, 2008)

Freeing Your Child from OCD: A Powerful, Practical Program for Parents of Children and Adolescents by Tamar E. Chansky (Three Rivers Press, 2001)

Helping Your Child with OCD: A Workbook for Parents of Children with Obsessive Compulsive Disorder by Lee Fitzgibbons and Cherry Pedrick (New Harbinger Publications, 2003)

The Boy Who Couldn't Stop Washing: The Experience and Treatment of OCD by Judith L. Rapoport (Signet, 1991)

Tormenting Thoughts and Secret Rituals: The Hidden Epidemic of OCD by Ian Osborn (Dell, 1999)

What to do When Your Child Has OCD: Strategies and Solutions by Aureen Pinto Wagner (Lighthouse Press, 2002)

OCD: Help for Children and Adolescents by Mitzi Waltz (Patient Centered Guides, 2000)

For School Personnel:

Cognitive Behavioral Interventions in Educational Settings: A Handbook for Practice by Rosemary Mennuti, Arthur Freeman, and Ray W. Christner (Routledge, 2005)

For Clergy:

Obsessive-Compulsive Disorder: A guide for Family, Friends, and Pastors by Robert M. Collie (Routledge, 2005)

The Doubting Disease: Help for Scrupulosity and Religious Compulsions by Joseph W. Ciarrocchi (Paulist Press, 1995)

The Obsessive-Compulsive Disorder: Pastoral Care for The Road to Change by Robert M. Collie (Routledge, 2000)

Self-Help:
The OCD Workbook: Your Guide to Breaking Free From OCD by Bruce M. Hyman and Cherry Pedrick (New Harbinger Publications, 2005)

Getting Control: Overcoming Your Obsessions and Compulsions by Lee Baer (Plume, 2000)

Overcoming Obsessive Thoughts by Christine Purdon and David Clark (New Harbinger Publications, 2005)

Hair Pulling (Trichotillomania):
Help for Hair Pullers: Understanding and Coping with Trichotillomania by Nancy J. Keuthen, Dan J. Stein, and Gary A. Christenson (New Harbinger Publications, 2001)

The Hair-Pulling Problem: A Complete Guide to Trichotillomania by Fred Penzel (Oxford University Press, 2003)

Body Dysmorphic Disorder (BDD):
The BDD Workbook by James Claiborn and Cherry Pedrick (New Harbinger Publications, 2002)

Feeling Good About the Way You Look: A Program for Overcoming Body Image Problems by Sabine Wilhelm (The Guilford Press, 2006)

The Broken Mirror by Katharine A. Phillips (Oxford University Press, 2005)

Hoarding:
Overcoming Compulsive Hoarding by Fugen Neziroglu, Jerome Bubrick, and Jose Yaryura-Tobias (New Harbinger Publications, 2004)

Buried in Treasures: Help for Compulsive Acquiring, Saving, and Hoarding by David F. Tolin, Randy O. Frost, and Gail S. Steketee (Oxford University Press, 2007)

Bad Thoughts:
The Imp of the Mind by Lee Baer (Dutton Adult, 2002)</BL>

For Scrupulosity:
Scrupulous Anonymous by Reverend Thomas M. Santa (monthly newsletter)
http://mission.liguori.org/newsletters/scrupanon.htm

Movies:
As Good As It Gets (TriStar, 1997)
Look on Google and at YouTube and type "OCD." You will see that you are not alone.

Legal Issues and Advocacy:

Americans with Disabilities Act: United States Department of Justice
www.usdoj.gov

Individuals with Disabilities Education Act (IDEA): United States Department
of Education
www.ed.gov/offices/OSERS/Policy/IDEA/

For information on finding help for students with learning disabilities and
ADHD: www.collegeboard.com/disable/counsel/html/indx000.html.

About Homework:

*Homework Success for Children with ADHD: A Family–School Intervention
    Program* by Thomas J. Power, James L. Karustis, Dina F. Habboushe Harth,
    and Dina F. Habboushe (The Guilford Press, 2001)

Glossary

A

Addiction: A pattern of drug abuse characterized by compulsive use of the drug, excessive focus on getting a supply of the drug, and a high likelihood of relapse when the drug use is stopped.

Adrenergic: Having to do with nerve pathways in which the neurotransmitters involved are epinephrine (adrenaline) or norepinephrine.

Adrenaline: A hormone secreted into the body that stimulates physiology that deals with fear and anxiety. Also called epinephrine.

Adverse event: (also called side effect) Any unwanted and undesirable action of a drug.

Affect: One's emotional tone; if sustained it becomes mood.

Agonist: A medication that has the same action as the natural neurotransmitter (e.g., a medication that has similar effects to epinephrine).

Agoraphobia: Fear of going outside or being in open or public places.

Anorexia nervosa: An eating disorder characterized by low body weight and body image distortion with an obsessive fear of gaining weight.

Antibody: One of many proteins found on a particular type of white blood cell (B cell); is secreted into the blood or elsewhere after a stimulus (e.g., presence of bacteria).

Antidepressants: Medicines used to stop depression; they are non-addictive (e.g., SSRIs like Prozac, TCAs like Anafranil).

Antipsychotics: See neuroleptics.

Anxiety attack: An episode of fear that is not as defined as a panic attack and does not have to occur out of the blue, as most panic attacks do, but may have a known trigger.

Anxiolytics: Type of medication that combats anxiety.

Asperger syndrome: One of several autism spectrum disorders (ASD) characterized by difficulties in social interaction and by restricted, stereotyped patterns of behavior, interests, and activities. Asperger syndrome is distinguished from the other ASDs in presenting no general delay in language or cognitive development.

Augmentation strategies: Used in clinical practice when patients fail to achieve remission on one medicine. At that point, another medicine may be added to increase the action of the first one.

Autism: A brain development disorder that impairs social interaction and communication; causes restricted and repetitive behavior, all starting before a child is 3 years old.

Autosomal dominant transmission: In genetics and heredity, a trait that needs to be in only one parent to be transmitted to the offspring.

B

Basal ganglia: Also referred to as the striatum. A group of interconnected nuclei that lies deep within the brain and includes the caudate, putamen, globus pallidus, and the thalamus. Each of the nuclei (and its connections to other brain structures) appears to be involved in certain disorders, like ADHD, tics, Parkinson disease, and chorea.

Behavioral therapy: A type of non-drug treatment aimed at changing overt behavior by a variety of techniques, such as systematic desensitization, relaxation training, flooding, participant modeling, and positive and negative reinforcement.

Benzodiazepines: A type of drug used for short-term treatment of panic attacks to decrease anxiety; potentially addictive.

Bipolar disorder: A mood disorder where the person experiences both an elated state (hypomania or mania) and at other times depression.

Body dysmorphic disorder (BDD): A preoccupation with imagined defects in appearance; the concern is excessive and causes distress in social situations.

Bulimia nervosa: An eating disorder in which patients are obsessed about weight, binge on food and then purge (vomiting or laxative use), or use excessive exercise to achieve their concept of thin.

C

Catecholamine: A group of neurotransmitters that includes dopamine, epinephrine, and norepinephrine.

Caudate: Nucleus within the basal ganglia that is rich in dopamine. It appears to be involved in ADHD, and it is smaller in children with ADHD.

Cerebrospinal fluid: Fluid that surrounds and fills the spaces within the brain and the spinal cord; also found in the spaces around nerve cells in the brain that neurotransmitters pass through.

Chorea: Rapid, jerky, involuntary, irregular muscle movements or twitching.

Cingulate gyrus: The medial part of the brain. It partially wraps around the corpus callosum. It functions as an integral part of the limbic system, which is involved with emotion formation and processing, learning, and memory.

Clinical trial: A carefully monitored study of a drug or a treatment using a drug that involves a large group of people with the goal of testing that drug's effectiveness and safety.

Cognitive: Pertaining to cognition, the process of being aware, knowing, thinking, learning, and judging.

Cognitive-behavioral therapy (CBT): A psychotherapy based on cognition (awareness), assumptions, beliefs, evaluations, and behaviors. Therapeutic techniques vary within the different approaches to CBT, according to the particular client or issue, but commonly include keeping a diary of significant events and associated feelings, thoughts, and behaviors. Varieties of CBT include dialectical behavior therapy, cognitive therapy, cognitive behavior modification, and exposure and response prevention, and multimodal therapy.

Cognitive therapy (CT): A type of psychotherapy in which the therapist seeks to identify and change distorted or unrealistic ways of thinking, and therefore to influence emotion and behavior.

Comorbid: When two disorders exist at the same time in the same individual.

Compulsions: Repetitive behaviors or mental acts that a person feels driven to perform in response to an obsession, or according to internal rules that must be applied rigidly.

Conditioning: The process of acquiring, developing, educating, establishing, learning, or training new responses in an individual.

Conduct disorder: Disorder in which there is an active transgression of societal rules.

Corpus callosum: A structure that lies between the left and right brain hemispheres and is required for passing information between them. It tends to be smaller than normal in children with ADHD.

D

Delusion: A fixed, false belief.

Depression: A state of lowered mood, usually with disturbances of sleep, appetite, suicidal thoughts, and so forth.

Diagnostic and Statistical Manual of Mental Disorders, Fourth Edition (DSM-IV-TR): Reference textbook of classifications used by mental health professionals to diagnose people with mental disorders.

Dopamine: A hormone and neurotransmitter. Dopamine cannot cross the blood–brain barrier; thus, when given as a drug, it does not directly affect the central nervous system. L-DOPA (levodopa), which is the precursor (chemical that the body converts to the active drug) of dopamine, can be given because it can cross the blood–brain barrier and affect the central nervous system. Dopamine is a precursor to norepinephrine (noradrenaline) and then epinephrine (adrenaline).

Drug (or drug–drug) interaction: When two or more drugs are given together and interfere with each other, possibly producing side effects or decreasing the effectiveness of one or more of the drugs.

Dysmorphic: An abnormality of the structure of a part of the body.

Dystonia: A brain disease in which muscles contract and produce repetitive, irregular spasms and twisting or abnormal postures.

E

Echocardiogram: An ultrasound record of the heart.

Efficacy: Effectiveness.

Ego: The self, a conscious part of the mind.

Ego-dystonic: Behaviors that are in conflict with the ego—i.e., in conflict with a person's ideal self-image.

Ego-syntonic: Behaviors consistent with one's ideal self-image.

Electrocardiogram (EKG): An electrical record of the heart that shows the heart's electrical currents; useful test to diagnose certain cardiovascular problems or disease.

Electroencephalogram (EEG): A test that measures brain electrical activity and is particularly useful in looking for seizure disorders.

Enzyme: A protein that speeds up a chemical reaction in a living organism.

Epinephrine: (also called adrenaline) A hormone released in the body after a stress stimulus. It is a "fight or flight" chemical that enables a person to flee or fight an enemy or danger.

Exposure and response prevention (ERP): A treatment method available from behavioral psychologists and cognitive-behavioral therapists for a variety of anxiety disorders; based on the idea that a therapeutic effect is achieved as subjects confront their fears and discontinue their escape response.

Executive functioning: Abilities, located in the frontal lobes, which draw upon more fundamental or primary cognitive skills, such as attention, language, and perception, to generate higher level of creative and abstract thought.

F

Food and Drug Administration (FDA): The U.S. federal agency that regulates drugs, devices, and food. In Canada, the equivalent is "Health Canada."

Frontal cortex: Front section of the brain that controls planning, organizing, starting, persisting, shifting, and inhibiting impulsive behaviors.

Frontostriatal circuit: The connections between the frontal lobes of the brain and the basal ganglia that are located deeper within the brain.

Functional imaging (fMRI): MRI of the brain done while an activity is being performed and that will show where that activity is happening.

G

GABA system: The system of neurotransmitters in various parts of the brain that are responsible for inhibiting neurons. If the GABA system is not working well, nerve cells are not turned off (inhibited) when they should be, and excess stimulation can occur that results in panic attacks and other unwanted events (see gamma aminobutyric acid).

Gamma aminobutyric acid (GABA): The most abundant central nervous system amino acid; works to inhibit neuronal transmission. It may malfunction in panic disorders.

Gene: A DNA sequence that codes for a protein. Genes are the biological basis of heredity.

Generalized anxiety disorder (GAD): A constant, excessive worry with restlessness, fatigue, irritability, and sleep disturbances; GAD patients can also experience their minds going blank, muscle tension, and feeling on edge.

Generic medication: A drug that contains the same active ingredient(s) as the name brand, though the inactive ingredients (e.g., fillers), shape, color, preservatives, and packaging may be different. In many instances, generics are just as good as the name brand and cost less. But some people do notice a difference and need the name brand in order to feel like they are getting the same amount of medication each dose/day.

Glutamate: Glutamate is the most abundant excitatory neurotransmitter in the mammalian nervous system. Because of its role in synaptic plasticity, it is believed that glutamic acid is involved in cognitive functions like learning and memory in the brain.

H

Half life: A measure of the duration of a drug's action; how long it takes before one-half the dose is gone from the body. Drugs with long half lives can be given infrequently, whereas drugs with short half lives need to be given frequently.

Hallucination: The apparent, often strong subjective perception of an object or event when no such stimulus or situation is present; may be visual, auditory, tactile, or involve smell or taste sensations.

Hippocampus: A region of the temporal lobe of the brain that controls learning and memory.

Hoarding: The excess storing of food, money, or other goods.

Hyperthyroidism: Increased thyroid hormone secretion causing such symptoms as anxiety and weight loss; sometimes can mimic panic attacks.

Hypochondriasis (hypochondria): A condition in which a healthy person believes and worries that he or she is ill.

Hypothalamus: An area of the brain below the thalamus involved in the control of the nervous system and certain hormones.

I

Id: The unorganized part of the personality structure that contains the basic drives. The id is unconscious (as per Freud's original description).

Incidence: The number of cases or events per time period (for example, 100 new cases of infection per year in a town).

Insight: The ability to recognize one's own mental illness or mental state. An insight is the derivation of a rule that links cause with effect.

L

Labeling: When referring to a drug, the FDA-approved documentation describing the use, dose, side effects, warnings, etc., for a drug

Limbic system: Brain structures, including the hypothalamus, responsible for the sense of smell, emotions, and behavior.

M

Magnetic resonance imaging (MRI): A technique that creates 3-dimensional images of brain structures using strong magnetic fields. It does not involve x-rays.

Metabolism: The body's reaction to a medication; faster in some than in others. Thus, people can require different doses of the same medication to receive similar effects.

Monoamine oxidase inhibitors (MAOIs): A standard medication for panic attacks. They work by stopping the breakdown of monoamines (like serotonin and norepinephrine) by irreversibly inhibiting the enzyme monoamine oxidase.

N

Neuroleptics: (also called antipsychotics) A group of psychoactive drugs commonly, but not exclusively used to treat psychosis. Antipsychotics are broadly divided into two groups, the typical or first-generation antipsychotics and the atypical or second-generation antipsychotics.

Neurological: Refers to functions controlled by the brain.

Neuron: A nerve cell, which is the basic cell unit of the brain and spinal cord. It can send and receive information from other brain cells.

Neuropsychological assessment: Series of tests used to examine the behavioral expression of brain function.

Neuroreceptor: A structural protein molecule on the nerve cell that binds to a specific factor, such as a neurotransmitter.

Neurotransmitter: Upon stimulus, a chemical agent that is released by a nerve cell (the presynaptic nerve cell) and travels through the space between that cell and the next nerve cell (synapse) to the postsynaptic cell, where it either stimulates or suppresses that cell. Dopamine, serotonin, and norepinephrine are neurotransmitters.

Non-selective serotonin uptake inhibitor (NSRI): A drug used in the treatment of OCD. An example is clomipramine (Anafranil). These drugs inhibit more than one neurotransmitter uptake whereas selective serotonin uptake inhibitors only work against the neurotransmitter serotonin and not the others.

Noradrenaline (or norepinephrine): A catecholamine hormone secreted from the adrenal gland, similar to adrenaline but having different effects on bronchial (lung) smooth muscle and the heart.

Nucleus: A central nervous system structure that is composed mainly of gray matter and that acts as transit point for electrical signals.

O

Obsessions: Recurrent and persistent thoughts, impulses, or images that are experienced as intrusive and inappropriate and that cause marked anxiety or distress.

Obsessive-compulsive disorder: A mental disorder that involves obsessions (thoughts, images, or impulses that occur over and over and feel out of control, which the person finds disturbing and intrusive and which do not make sense) and compulsions (certain acts that are done over and over again according to "rules"; these rituals are performed to obtain relief from the discomfort caused by obsessions).

Occipital lobe: Rear section of the brain that controls vision.

P

Parietal lobe: Midsection of the brain that controls sensory functions and also serves to integrate several brain functions simultaneously, such as seeing and hearing.

PANDAS: An abbreviation for pediatric autoimmune neuropsychiatric disorders associated with streptococcal infections. This diagnosis is used to describe a set of children thought to have a rapid onset of OCD and/or tic disorders such as Tourette syndrome, following group A beta-hemolytic streptococcal (GABHS) infections such as "strep throat" and scarlet fever.

Panic attack: A sudden, discrete period of intense anxiety, with physiological arousal.

Paraphilia: A recurring sexual impulse or behavior to objects such as fabrics, designs, or feet.

Phobia: An objectively unfounded, morbid dread or fear that arouses a state of panic; used in combination with the object that inspires the fear such as "agoraphobia."

Placebo reaction: When a person has a positive effect from an innocuous substance such as a sugar pill.

Positron emission tomography (PET) Scan: A test in which a small amount of radioactive glucose (sugar) is injected into a vein, and a scanner is used to make detailed, computerized pictures of areas inside the body (e.g., the brain) where the glucose is used.

Postsynaptic neuron Receives the message carried by the neurotransmitter.

Post-traumatic Stress Disorder (PTSD): An anxiety disorder that can develop after exposure to one or more terrifying events that threatened or caused grave physical harm. It is a severe and ongoing emotional reaction to an extreme psychological trauma.

Presynaptic neuron: Sends the message by releasing a neurotransmitter.

Prevalence: The total number of cases of a disease in a population at a particular point in time. This number includes new and old cases (e.g., the prevalence in our town of this disease was nine cases per million people in May, 2009).

Prophylactic: Prevention of a disease or process that can lead to a disease.

Psychiatrist: A medical doctor (MD) specializing in the treatment of mental diseases and disorders. Psychiatrists are legally permitted to prescribe medications.

Psychologist: A professional with a PhD who can provide behavioral and other types of therapy and can administer and analyze psychological tests, but cannot prescribe medication (see psychiatrist).

Psychopharmacologist: Psychiatrist who specializes in medication treatment for mental disorders.

Psychosis: Loss of contact with reality. People with psychosis may have one or more of the following hallucinations, delusions, thought disorder, or lack of insight. The symptoms are similar in nature to mental confusion and delirium.

Psychosocial: The impact of social situations and mental health upon each other.

Putamen: A portion of the basal ganglia that forms the outermost part of the lenticular nucleus; appears to play a role in reinforcement learning.

R

Rebound irritability: Moodiness, fatigue seen as a medication is stopped and wears off.

Receptor: A protein molecule on the surface of a cell that receives and binds neurotransmitters, hormones, etc.

Receptor sites: Places on neurons that bind neurotransmitters or where the medications act. Some medications can increase or decrease the number or sensitivity of receptors.

Recovery: Full recovery is defined as an almost complete and objective disappearance of symptoms and corresponds to a Y-BOCS score of <8 for OCD.

Remission: When symptoms are reduced to a minimal level, with a Y-BOCS of <16. Recovery and remission are considered high levels of response.

Residual symptoms: Symptoms that persist even when treatment has been received at a good therapeutic dose and for the usual length of time usually needed.

Rett syndrome: An inherited, X-linked neurological disorder that is fatal to males. In females, there is rapid neurological deterioration leading to dementia, autism, and loss of speech and voluntary movements.

Reversible inhibitor of monoamine oxidase (RIMA): A medication that allows the enzyme monomine oxidase to be reversibly inhibited; that is, if the enzyme needs to be used, then the MAOI will bounce off and allow the breakdown of monoamines, such as tyramine. Tyramine can cause the release of stored monoamines, such as dopamine, norepinephrine, and epinephrine.

Ritual: A repetitive, systematic behavioral process enacted to neutralize or prevent anxiety; a symptom of obsessive-compulsive disorder (OCD).

S

Schizophrenia: A psychiatric disorder characterized by psychosis with delusions and hallucinations.

School phobia: Excessive social anxiety (anxiety in social situations) causing abnormally considerable distress and impaired ability to function in at least some areas of daily life.

Selective serotonin reuptake inhibitor (SSRI): A type of antidepressant that does not allow serotonin to be taken up again by neuroreceptors, thereby causing more serotonin to be present to the neurons, which decreases panic attacks; includes drugs such as Prozac, Zoloft, Paxil, Celexa, Luvox, and Lexapro.

Separation anxiety: A psychological condition in which an individual has excessive anxiety regarding separation from home or from people to whom the individual has a strong emotional attachment (like a father and mother).

Serotonin: A neurotransmitter that may be decreased in depression and panic attacks.

Serotonin reuptake inhibitors (SRIs): Drugs that increase the level of serotonin in the synapses but are not selective and have some actions on other neurotransmitters as well. They are used in the treatment of OCD and other disorders like depression.

Social phobia: A marked and persistent fear of one or more social or performance situations, exposure to unfamiliar people, or to possible scrutiny by others. The person fears acting in an anxious way that will be embarrassing or humiliating.

Social worker: A healthcare professional who can provide behavioral and other types of psychotherapy but cannot prescribe medication (see psychiatrist, psychologist). Treatment focus can be on the whole individual as well as family and/or groups.

Striatum: Part of the basal ganglia that consists of several interconnected regions/nuclei deep within the brain, specifically the caudate and the putamen.

Subclinical: A condition or disease that shows no signs or symptoms and is detectable only by special tests.

Synapse: The fluid-filled space between two neurons (brain cells) where neurotransmitters can pass from one cell to the next.

Synaptic plasticity: The ability of the connection between two nerves to change in strength. Thus the response of a receptor neuron to a neurotransmitter may not always be the same. It may be stronger or weaker.

T

Tachycardia: A fast heartbeat.

Temporal lobe: Lower section of the brain that controls memory and language comprehension.

Temporal lobe epilepsy: Epilepsy in which epileptic origins are located in the temporal lobe of the brain.

Thalamus: A part of the brain that has to do with pain and some emotions.

Tics: Involuntary muscle movements or twitches or vocal outbursts.

Tourette syndrome A disorder characterized by numerous motor and vocal tics. To be diagnosed with Tourette syndrome, tics must be present for at least 1 year.

Treatment response: A reduction of 25% to 35% of the Y-BOCS score.

Trichotillomania: Hair pulling.

Tricyclic antidepressants (TCAs): Among the first types of medication used to treat depression; popular before SSRIs came into wide use; can be used to treat panic disorder.

Twins: Two offspring resulting from the same pregnancy, either of the same or opposite sex. Dizygotic twins (commonly known as fraternal twins, but also referred to as non-identical twins or biovular twins), like any other siblings, have an extremely small chance of having the exact same chromosome profile. Monozygotic twins, frequently referred to as identical twins, occur when a single egg is fertilized to form one zygote (monozygotic) that then divides into two separate embryos. Their traits and physical appearances are not exactly the same; although they have nearly identical DNA.

V

Vocal tics: Involuntary sounds such as throat clearing, sniffing, or words.

W

Withdrawal: The psychological and or physical reaction to abruptly stopping a dependence-producing drug.

Y

Yale-Brown Obsessive compulsive Scale (Y-BOCS): A test to rate the severity of OCD symptoms and to monitor improvement during treatment.

Index